TEACHING THE WORLD TO SLEEP

TEACHING THE WORLD
TO SLEEP

Psychological and Behavioural Assessment
and Treatment Strategies for People with
Sleeping Problems and Insomnia

David R. Lee

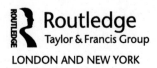

Routledge
Taylor & Francis Group

LONDON AND NEW YORK

First published in 2017 by Karnac Books Ltd

Published 2018 by Routledge
2 Park Square, Milton Park, Abingdon, Oxon, OX14 4RN
711 Third Avenue, New York, NY 10017, USA

Routledge in an imprint of the Taylor & Francis Group, an informa business

British Library Cataloguing in Publication Data

A C.I.P. for this book is available from the British Library

ISBN-13: 9781782203452 (pbk)

Typeset by V Publishing Solutions Pvt Ltd., Chennai, India

CONTENTS

v

LIST OF FIGURES

ACKNOWLEDGEMENTS AND THANKS

Thanks and love go to my Mum and Dad for all their love and support, over all the years.

For their untiring patience and support, much thanks and love go to: Mel, Henry, Cara, Cameron, and Michael.

Thanks also to my partners in spreading the word Vicki Gilman, Mandy Martell, Ben Hope, Jade Warner, and Dr. Melanie Davis.

Thanks also go out to Professors Colin Espie, Allison Harvey, and Kevin Morgan for their permissions to reproduce materials in this publication.

Finally, thanks go to all at Karnac Books and especially to Rod Tweedy, Oliver Rathbone, and Constance Govindin for their helpful guidance and support throughout the preparation of this book.

This first half of this book was written at The Riverhouse, and the second half at The Summerhouse, both in Shotley Bridge, in the tranquil and beautiful surroundings of County Durham between February 2015 and February 2016 (some of it was also written on multiple, lengthy train journeys around the country, whilst spreading the word).

ABOUT THE AUTHOR

David Lee, BSc, PhD, CertEd, CPsychol, AFBPsS ,CSci, is a chartered psychologist and chartered scientist who has been teaching, researching, and disseminating findings from his own research into sleep and the psychobehavioural treatment of insomnia for the last fifteen years. He holds memberships with the World Association of Sleep Medicine, the British Sleep Society, The Association of Personal Injury Lawyers, The British Association of Behavioural and Cognitive Psychotherapists and The British Psychological Society, where he also holds an associate fellowship. He has held various academic posts, but now works full-time as Clinical Director for Sleep Unlimited Ltd. A company which specialises in the delivery of training of psychobehavioural treatment strategies for insomnia under the umbrella of the REST programme (described fully in Chapter Five), and in the assessment and treatment of individuals with insomnia. The company is increasingly working with legal firms, case managers and multi-disciplinary teams; providing expert and treatment reports for people who have experienced head injuries, and clinical negligence casework.

INTRODUCTION

What this book is about

There is myriad information published in the area of sleep and any book on the subject will naturally be required to be somewhat selective in the material presented within its pages. The specific audiences to whom this book is aimed are described in the following section, but by way of an introduction to this book its contents will be briefly summarised here.

After an initial inspection of the existing scientific background to what is known (and still remains to be studied) about sleep in the second chapter, subsequent chapters will, by turn, examine: insomnia and the parasomnias in Chapter Two; the assessment and treatment of sleep problems in Chapters Four and Five, respectively; before describing current, state-of-the art psychobehavioural treatment strategies currently recommended as a first line therapy for the treatment of the person with insomnia in Chapter Five. Following this, attention is then focused on more vulnerable client groups in Chapter Six and the book concludes with a brief examination of the background theory and clinical applications of dreams and "dreamwork" in the therapeutic setting in Chapter Seven.

Who this book is for

This book has evolved from a series of lectures, workshops, and seminars that have been delivered by the author to a wide range of audiences over the last decade or so. The audiences to which these presentations have been delivered fall, broadly speaking, into two groups; and it is to those groups that this book has been designed, and to whom it is aimed.

The first group are people who do not sleep well. They may not sleep well for a number of reasons: their sleep problem may be a recent, or an enduring problem for them; they often have on-going problems with their sleep despite engagement with health services; and so have been drawn to attend the author's presentations and engage his services to assist with the treatment of their insomnia. This book is written to be accessible to this group of people and Chapters Two, Five, and Six will be of particular note to these readers.

The second group broadly comprises the population of "healthcare professionals". The list is long, but predominantly includes (in no particular order): psychologists (clinical, educational, occupational, and forensic), psychotherapists (of various discipline), counsellors, nurses, midwives, physicians, general practitioners, psychiatrists, physiotherapists, occupational therapists, and solicitors, lawyers, and barristers who work in the medico-legal domain. To this group of readers then the whole book will have utility. The ambition of this book for this group is that the assessment forms and psychobehavioural treatment information contained in these pages will be of particular use in practicing with, and supporting their clients who are experiencing problems with their sleep.

CHAPTER ONE

The science of sleep

There have been many books written about sleep, the varying theories about its nature and purpose, informed from multiple angles (adults, infants, animals, and even plants!) over many decades. As stated in the introduction, the purpose of this book is to deliver information that is current and state-of-the-art: to people with insomnia to help improve their sleep experience; and to healthcare practitioners in order to inform and enhance their practice. As a result, this chapter will not engage in a lengthy repetition of the evolving theories as to the purpose of sleep over the years, but will describe where we are at the moment and how this can be of use to the individual with a sleep problem and the practicing healthcare professional, restricting its range to human sleep in health and "disease". This chapter is subdivided into sections that will examine our current knowledge about sleep from different perspectives. After an initial examination of the various states of consciousness, we will look at circadian rhythms, sleep stages, current ideas about memory, how sleep changes as we age, the influence of light on our sleep, tiredness, how social cues impact on our sleep, and then how physical and psychological insults can reduce the quality and quantity of our sleep. This chapter will then conclude by pulling all these elements together to explain the complex and dynamic nature of sleep. After reading through this chapter it is anticipated that the reader will have a good base-knowledge about the science underpinning what it is to sleep in health and in poor health, so providing them with a good foundation on which to introduce therapeutic interventions to help improve sleep in themselves, and for their families, friends, and clients.

States of consciousness

So to begin with it is worth looking at our minds and how we live life as perceived by our brains. Essentially there are three states of consciousness, which are all very different from one another; and our brains shift between these states continuously throughout our lives, every day, all the time. If we do not allow this shifting to occur, we suffer. If anyone has stayed awake for more than a couple of days and nights, then they will be acutely aware of what this feels like. Jet lag, shift work, being a new parent, there are many ways to experience these feelings, in fact *everyone* knows the feeling, we call it "tired", we call it "fatigued". This is because we need to shift our consciousness regularly, as to exactly *why* we need to do this still remains something of an enigma, although we are becoming increasingly aware these days that it has something very important to do with memory (to be discussed later in this chapter). The consequences of not shifting are serious, from mild discomfort, to billions of lost working hours (and so money), and huge industrial accidents with major consequences to people, economies, and the environment. The big things we have all seen on the news—Chernobyl nuclear power plant disaster, the Exxon-Valdes oil tanker spillage, the Three Mile Island nuclear core melt down, the Challenger space shuttle explosion, and so on. The smaller, subtler impact of mild to moderate tiredness and fatigue on the population is much more difficult to measure, but estimates are massive. In the US, where there have been detailed investigations conducted into the cost insomnia to society indicate direct cost estimates of fourteen billion dollars annually, rising to $100 billion for indirect costs (including work-related accidents and lost productivity), these were estimates from early in this second millennium (Sivertsen & Nordhus, 2007).

So what are these three states? First—we are awake, our brains are mildly to hugely active and we are "conscious", we have volition, we are in control. Our attention is malleable and we range from "alpha" type activity (for example: zoning out in front of the television; or driving home from work and not really remembering the journey). Alpha states are where our brains could quite easily slip into another state of consciousness, the opposite end of the wakefulness spectrum is occupied by gamma wave activity. Gamma is where we are super-alert, and the best way to get our brains into this state is to play a team game like football where we are paying attention to ourselves, our team, the opposition, the ball, the opposition's goal, our goal, who to pass to, where to run etc., playing 3D "Shoot-em-up" maze games on computer consoles has a similar effect. State one is conscious, awake, aware, and in control; but every twenty-four hours we need to spend a significant proportion of time (between a quarter and a third of the time for most adults) in the two other states which occur during sleep. Namely REM and non-REM sleep.

Sleep, in many ways, is the opposite of being awake. We are not aware, we cannot shift our attention (with the exception of a few people who experience "lucid" dreams, but even then that ability to shift attention is quite limited), and we are "unconscious". Different parts of our brains go quiet or acquiesce, while other parts become more active, and we are beginning to get an understanding as to why, particularly with advances in functional Magnetic Resonance Imaging (fMRI) techniques. More on this later. REM sleep, as most people are probably aware, stands for Rapid Eye Movement sleep and our sleep period shifts between REM and non-REM sleep in a ninety-minute cycle (in the adult human), we will talk more about this "circadian" rhythm of the REM—non-REM cycle in the next section. Again, why we cycle between these other two states of consciousness whilst asleep is still something of a mystery, but we will look at some possible explanations for this later on.

If we take a look at Figure 1 (below) we can see a graphical representation of the electrical activity of our brains in these three states of consciousness. "Awake" is characterised by high frequency, but low amplitude (or height of the wave) waveforms—the higher the frequency, the more "awake" we are, so gamma activity is very fast, beta waves are intermediate and alpha relatively slow waveforms; and that makes sense if we think about how active our waking brains are when we are engaged in different activities. As our brains tire and get ready for sleep we lose the higher frequencies and become more alpha dominated. We know what this "drifting off" feels like, because we do it every night and have done so, every night, for the whole of our lives. It is very difficult to go to sleep if we are very excited (i.e., our brains are banging away at a high frequency). So gradually our brainwaves slow down, we "phase-out", we "drift-off" and this (electrically speaking) is our brainwaves slowing and the amplitude (height) of the brainwaves increasing. We have entered stage one non-REM sleep—also referred to as transitional sleep. This stage is not regarded as true sleep, but an interface period between wakefulness and sleep. This stage is characterised by alpha waves and some theta wave activity, but a loss of the higher gamma and beta frequencies. We spend a very little time in this stage, but some interesting things can occur to us during this time. We can twitch and jerk ourselves back to wakefulness here (so-called hypnic jerks); our arms and legs can feel heavy, twitch, and feel uncomfortable (restless legs syndrome (RLS), and periodic limb movements (PLM)) can also occur here; and we can have, sometimes vivid, visual experiences: hypnogogic (going to sleep) and hypnopompic (leaving sleep) hallucinations. Usually though, we pass through this stage relatively quickly and without incident into stage two non-REM sleep, the lightest stage of true sleep. This stage is again characterised by a reduction in the frequency and an increase in the amplitude of the brain's electrical waveforms, but is identified by the appearance of K-Complexes and Spindles (see Figure 1 below), and by a loss of alpha and a predominance of theta wave activity. These K complexes and spindles are enigmatic in their own right with uncertainty about their true function, but they are probably resultant from brainstem control mechanisms that may serve as an external noise suppression feature to allow us to maintain sleep and progress into our deeper "restorative" sleep. These deeper stages three and four of non-REM sleep are collectively known as deep sleep, delta wave sleep, or slow wave sleep (SWS) the latter being the most popular (Rechtschaffen & Kales, 1968). Recently stages three and four have been grouped together and we now refer to stage three only as SWS.

Slow wave sleep is again characterised by a reduction in the frequency and an increase in the amplitude of the brain's electrical wave activity. If one compares these waves to those characteristic of wakefulness in Figure 1 below there is a striking difference. These big, deep, and slow waves are the waves that we need to get every twenty-four hours to restore, refresh, and enable us to live functional lives. Without them we suffer the consequences, this kind of sleep is fundamental and we have got some pretty good evidence as to why. We will look into these after a quick word or two about REM sleep. So sleep stages one to three collectively comprise state of consciousness two—non-REM sleep.

State of consciousness three is REM sleep. REM looks like wakefulness (please see Figure 1 again), which is why it has sometimes been referred to as "paradoxical" sleep. If one just looks at the electrical activity of the brain (by sticking electrodes on top of the head and measuring the minute electrical activity of the brain's cortices through the scalp, (this form of assessment is referred to as the electroencephalogram or EEG) we see what looks like state one—wakefulness. However, if we place other electrodes (under the eyes and under the chin, the electro-occulogram and electromyogram respectively) we see rapid eye movements, hence REM, and a loss of muscle tone in the muscle under the chin. The placing of electrodes in an EEG, occulogram, and myogram combination is referred to as polysomnography and is the way sleep is measured in a sleep laboratory. There are sometimes other electrodes placed on limbs, respiratory and cardiac areas to measure other physiological responses too. The reason for the myogram electrode is to detect atonia, or paralysis. A key feature of healthy REM sleep is a loss of muscle tone. If you have ever woken up with a damp pillow, this is because you have been in REM, sleeping on your side and you have dribbled out of the side of your mouth as your jaw has slackened during REM periods. We are still not sure why this paralysis in REM occurs, but there are numerous theories, including: not acting out our dreams, reducing activity so we do not awaken and remain asleep etc. Indeed, the whole purpose and reason for REM remains largely debated with multiple theories abound as to the phenomenon. There are memory-related hypotheses, the central nervous system stimulation (ontogenetic hypothesis), scanning and sentinel (observing the environment for threat) hypotheses, and even a defensive immobilisation hypothesis, whereby we look as if we are dead and so are left alone by potential predators. It may well be that there is truth in a number, or even a combination, of these theories and we will return to one of the memory hypotheses later as this seems to have the most credibility and application in modern humans.

So there are the three states of consciousness, Awake, REM sleep and non-REM sleep. We will return to these ideas in further sections of this chapter to fill out on the current thinking as to purposes of the sleep states, and their significance to the primary state of wakefulness, which affects us all. Before this though, we will take a brief look at the circadian rhythm.

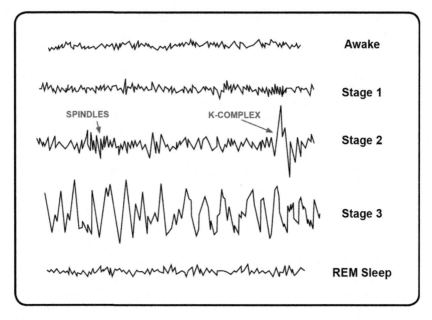

Figure 1. Electrical waveforms of the three states of consciousness.

Circadian rhythms

There is a clock inside our brains, which operates continuously and without our conscious awareness, controlling a whole range of our physiological functions. This clock is not exclusive to humans, all animals and even plants have "rhythmicity", periods of activity interspersed with regular periods of inactivity or quiescence. This rhythmicity was first noted as far back as 4BCE, but the first experimental evidence of their existence was conducted on plants in 1729 by a French scientist called Jean-Jacques d'Ortous de Mairan. Since then several periodicity genes have been identified, including: the CLOCK, PER1, PER2 and PER3 genes, simpler organisms have just one of these genes, more complex organisms have two, three, or all four of these genes, whose effect is to provide the host organism with this internal, or endogenous, clock. Humans have all three of the PER genes and the CLOCK gene and these are known to effect the suprachiasmatic nucleus (SCN) two distinctive groups of cells at the back of the hypothalamus in the centre of our brains. Adults have a circadian rhythm of ninety minutes, and this is very regular. Even in people in the advanced stages of dementia, this endogenous rhythm clicks along continuously and many of our functions are controlled and influenced by it. The cycling of REM and non-REM sleep follow this rhythm. Hunger and thirst, urine production, alertness, even creativity follow this rhythm, along with many other functions. Here are a couple of practical examples that help to explain the phenomenon: We are all familiar with a dip in alertness mid-afternoon, and another before we go to bed, at these times our circadian rhythm is reaching a minimum, our alertness is at its lowest, and it is here when we can easily initiate sleep. If we wait half an hour though, our alertness is on the rise and we begin to reach a peak, this is when sleep is very difficult to initiate. If you have ever shifted your bedtime from its normal time, then it is often difficult to get sleep. For example: "I'll be getting up early tomorrow to catch an early flight, so I'd better go to bed early," and then you cannot get off to sleep until the usual time. Or, you go to bed later than usual and think: "Why can't I sleep, it's past my usual bedtime, I should be tired and so I should be able to get to sleep". If you want to shift your bedtime from its usual slot then you need to move it by ninety minutes to catch the preceding, or succeeding, circadian dip. This can be hugely effective in the therapeutic intervention for insomnia and we will return to this later in Chapters Five and Six on the treatment of sleeping problems.

* * *

Another example of the circadian rhythm in action is something many people will be familiar with: the "Eureka moment". If you have ever found yourself "blocked", for example, you cannot think of an answer in an exam; or you cannot seem to find the right words to express yourself when writing something; or you are not performing to your usual standard in a certain task etc., then you are probably "dipping out" in your circadian rhythm. Leaving the task and returning to it forty-five minutes later and, suddenly, the answer is there, the words flow, the block has gone, the Eureka moment arrives—as your circadian rhythm is peaking. This is easy to see in action if you ever watch professional tennis matches, or snooker on the television. These matches are long in duration and so it is possible to observe individual players performing well, and then later they seem to go "off the boil". These fluctuations in performance are driven by the circadian rhythm. There is a large, unexplored opportunity to use the circadian rhythm to offset poor performance and optimise periods of high performance, not only in the

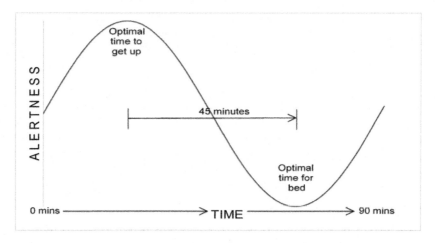

Figure 2. One cycle of the adult human circadian rhythm.

sports arena, but in all of our lives, both socially and professionally. Knowing your own rhythm and scheduling tasks and activities around it can enhance your performance and, perhaps more importantly, avoid tiredness-related errors and accidents.

Figure 2 above shows a simple illustration of one cycle of the circadian rhythm.

As mentioned above the circadian rhythm in adult humans has a period of ninety minutes, however, this is reduced in children and infants (Czeisler, Zimmerman, Ronda, Moore-Ede, & Weitzman, 1980). The very young have circadian rhythms of around forty-five–fifty minutes from birth and into the first year of life. The circadian rhythm then extends out in toddlers and young children to around sixty minutes, before extending out again to the ninety minute, adult period of ninety minutes around mid-childhood (Bes, Schulz, Navelet, & Salzarulo, 1991). The field of chronobiology is huge, but, for our purposes in this book, we will only refer to the circadian rhythm in its relationship to sleep. The following section examines the various sleep stages, the passage of which is determined by the circadian rhythm.

Sleep stages

As we saw in the first section of this chapter on the states of consciousness there are various sleep stages. REM sleep and non-REM sleep, which was divided into four stages and has, quite recently, been separated into three stages, combining stages three and four together (Iber, Ancoli-Israel, Chesson, & Quan, 2007). Stage one, or transitional sleep occupies the smallest amount of human sleep (about two–five per cent of sleep in the healthy adult). In health, wakefulness constitutes less than five per cent of the night, although much of this is beyond awareness (so-called microarousals which usually last less than a minute). Stage two sleep occupies around forty-five–fifty-five per cent of the night's sleep. Stage three was often regarded as a transitional phase between stages two and four (deep, slow wave sleep) and only occupies around three–eight per cent of the night's sleep. Stage four occupies around ten–fifteen per cent, leaving REM sleep occupying around twenty–twenty-five per cent of healthy adult sleep occurring to older criteria (Rechtschaffen & Kales, 1968). However, combining the deeper states of sleep together into stage three sleep following recent changes to the scoring guidelines, we now have approximately fifteen–twenty-five per cent of healthy adult sleep comprising slow wave sleep (Iber, Ancoli-Israel, Chesson, & Quan, 2007). These stages cycle in concert with the circadian rhythm of ninety minutes: REM to non-REM stages. The simplified hypnogram in Figure 3 shows this cycling, which follows the circadian rhythm (as described in the previous section), in healthy younger people and there are a few notable things to observe in this illustration.

Firstly, as we sleep we initially descend very quickly into a prolonged bout of deep, slow wave sleep (SWS), we then cycle up to our first bout of the night's REM sleep which is relatively short in duration before descending down again into another bout of SWS. This second bout of SWS is shorter than the first of the night, when we then cycle up again into another bout of REM sleep that is longer than the first REM bout of the night. This cycle repeats throughout the night, following (in the human adult) the ninety-minute circadian rhythm. What we see as the night progresses is: more SWS at the start of the night, that is replaced by more REM at the end of the night. This is true for all humans in health, at all ages and across both genders and all races. It is a phenomenon that is fundamental and universal.

All well and good, but which stage is the most important and why the cycling? If you deprive someone of their sleep for a few nights, they will obviously be very tired, and will sleep readily and for longer than usual afterwards to recover. Furthermore, there are a few, now

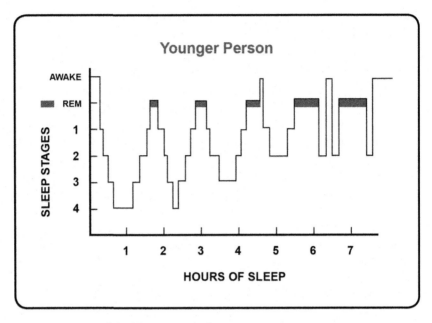

Figure 3. A simplified hypnogram from a typical younger person.

classic sleep deprivation studies, which have collectively answered this first question. These studies have all concurred that, after everywhere from mild to extreme sleep deprivation, recovery sleep is seen to have a large predominance of SWS at the expense of REM, and that REM is caught up on later, given the chance. The implication here is that SWS is more important than REM. Partial sleep deprivation studies (where participants have been allowed to sleep, but for a shorter time than usual) have shown that people can still function quite well on around four and a half hours of sleep (which is three ninety-minute REM/non-REM cycles). As we know that SWS predominates in the first few cycles of the night and that we can function quite well on shorter sleep, for a long time it was thought that REM was a kind of optional extra, designed to keep us sleeping, but not essential to our lives and psychological wellbeing (Åkerstedt, Kecklund, Ingre, Lekander, & Axelsson, 2009). We now know this not to be true, we do need REM sleep, and if you partially sleep deprive someone for a period of time they will not thank you for it, they will feel negative consequences of the experience, and they will revert back to their preferred sleep length (including some catch-up) after the period of partial sleep deprivation is over.

There is a classic sleep deprivation study which is worthy of mention here, not only because it was one of the first, but because of the seren-dipitous nature of it, and because of a number of important findings that we learned from this one single case. The unfortunately named Randy Gardner was a high school student in San Diego, California in the 1960s and, as part of a school-based science project, he decided to conduct an experiment on himself. He wondered what the effects of complete sleep deprivation would be on him mentally and physically. The first bit of serendipity—a really interesting idea. So, with the help of a couple of friends he stayed awake, mostly playing pinball in his garage. After a few days and nights attention to his experiment came to the attention of the local radio station which reported it to the local area, the second bit of serendipity. The third was that he happened to be living very close to a large naval base, on which was one of the real pioneers of sleep research, William Dement. Dement, who was working on the base at the time, heard about Randy's exploits and invited him to come onto the base where they would pay him to continue to stay awake; and so monitor the effects to inform how the serving forces would perform under conditions of deprived sleep (quite a common phenomenon on the battlefield). Of course Randy agreed. Then, after about four days and nights of no sleep, he went into Dement's lab on the naval base and began undergoing regular testing throughout the remainder of his record-breaking period of wakefulness. A few times during this period Randy got fed up and decided to quit, but he was encouraged to con-tinue by Dement with increased financial incentives. Eventually he did quit, after a quite amazing eleven days and eleven nights of total sleep deprivation, that is 264 hours, and remains a record. Although some have tried to repeat this and break the record, with others claiming they have bettered the 264 hours awake. These characters have not been able to substantiate their claims, so Randy still has the prize. The effects of this experience on Randy were not surprising, he felt as one would expect him to feel, but there were a few interesting things which emerged. He felt tired, obviously, he was also irritable, his performance on tests went up and down in concert with his circadian rhythm, and all of these were expected outcomes. He also became quite paranoid as time went on and experienced "mild peripheral visual hallucinations, problems with concentration and short-term memory," (Gulevich, Dement, &

Johnson, 1966) these findings were novel. However, the interesting outcomes really emerged after the sleep deprivation. Dement kept Randy on the base for a few days afterwards to monitor him and make sure he was alright, but also to examine how he recovered. Randy was usually a fairly normal sleeper, sleeping for around seven and a half to eight hours per night. On the first recovery night he slept for fourteen hours and forty minutes, the second night around ten and a half hours and then was back to his normal sleep length thereafter. He was again assessed at one, six, and ten weeks after the study and no detrimental effects of the sleep deprivation were noted, either psychologically or physically (Gulevich, Dement, & Johnson, 1966). This was quite radical, that someone could recover from such a huge disruption to their sleep so quickly, and that this recovery was complete. A note of caution here. Randy was a fit and healthy young man, and a willing volunteer. Many sleep studies have used students and younger people, in comfortable conditions, often with financial (and other, positive) incentives attached to such studies, and the collective conclusion has been that sleep deprivation has no long lasting negative physical or psychological impacts on such participants. This was picked up on by the Central Intelligence Agency who have justified sleep deprivation as a legitimate and ethical "interview" technique for use with enemies of the state as: "surprisingly, little seemed to go wrong with the subjects physically. The main effects lay with sleepiness and impaired brain functioning, but even these were no great cause for concern." From work reported by an experienced sleep researcher cited in a CIA memo on interrogation techniques (Bradbury, 2005). It should be very much noted here that sleep deprivation studies with willing volunteers in cosy sleep laboratories, with lots of fun stuff to do and with financial (or other, positive) incentives are a very different experience to being deprived of sleep in prison or detention, whilst under conditions of duress and distress. The two are simply not comparable. We now know that sleep deprivation in such conditions is extremely harmful and traumatising and we will look more on this later in this chapter in the section on psychological impacts.

Memory and schemas

To return to REM sleep and non-REM sleep for a moment, it is worth mentioning memory and the concept of a "forgettery". The first we are all familiar with, but the second is a relatively new idea, and we have got some evidence emerging that sleep is hugely important for both.

First, memory: there is a very small part of the brain, right in the centre near the hypothalamus, called the hippocampus. When we are in SWS the brain is quiet and acquiescing, with the exception of the hippocampus, which is fully awake, up and running, firing on all cylinders, and at its most active in the twenty-four-hour cycle. We know from a large number of studies that the hippocampus is critically important for the consolidation of memory, acting as a control centre in the middle of the brain, sending messages out into the cortices above it. Taxi drivers whom have learned all the streets in London, referred to as "doing the knowledge" have been shown to have larger hippocampi when training when compared to other people who have not had this training (Macguire et al., 2000). Chronic insomniacs have also been shown to have smaller hippocampi that normal sleepers (Riemann, Kloepfer, & Berger, 2009). These findings—and many others—have identified SWS as critical for the consolidation of memory. There is a useful analogy that can explain this a bit more. If you imagine that the inside of your head is a busy office, and that every thought that you have during the day generates a piece of paper in that office. During the course of a day we have many, many thoughts, about everything and anything. Some of those things are important, or even very important (e.g., I need to call the mortgage advisor), but other thoughts may be less so (e.g., which socks shall I wear today?; Ooh—look at that dirty car). But each of these generates a piece of paper. Then we sleep and our secretary (the hippocampus) comes into the office and starts to organise things. This organisation consists of sorting through all the paper and throwing out the rubbish (socks/dirty car); and prioritising the important things (sticking the "call the mortgage advisor" piece of paper on top of the in-tray for tomorrow morning) that is, encoding this into the cortex as something to be remembered and not forgotten. If we sleep well we will do a good job of organising our office and it will be tidy again by the morning, if we do not sleep well then the office will be a mess in the morning—this idea has important implications for our mental health and we will come back to this in the psychological impacts of sleep disturbance later in this chapter.

There is the analogy for SWS and the hippocampus, but we are still left standing a bit with where REM sleep fits into this picture. Some very recent work published in 2014 by Dieter Riemann,

Kai Speigelhalder, and colleagues from Freiberg in Germany (Landmann et al., 2014) has posited an advanced theory on the complex interplay between the memory, the forgettery, REM sleep, and SWS. Their work is highly innovative and at the cutting edge of our understanding of the psychophysiology of sleep in health, and how it changes in poor health. In order to explain this, we need to first examine the concept of schemas or frameworks. These will be familiar to many people, but, briefly for those unfamiliar with schemas another quick analogy.

If someone asks you to make them a cup of tea, and you have never done this before, it will be very difficult for you as you have had no experience in the task, no frame of reference, no "schema" for making tea. If you are then taught to do this, you will have a framework in your head for what (and how) it is to make tea. Once in place, you will then find it much easier to make, say, a cup of coffee, as you already have a very similar schema established in your mind for making tea. Once practiced at making tea and coffee, you will then find it quite easy to make any number of hot beverages (hot chocolate, herbal tea, chai etc.) as your framework for hot drinks is well established in your mind. We know from a large number of studies that learning is much improved after good sleep, and seriously impeded after poor sleep (and especially after no sleep). We are also pretty certain that this is why children need to sleep much more that adults. This is also thought to be why infants will need to be asleep and awake multiple times in a twenty-four-hour period as they have no schemas, and so need to assimilate much new information (and forget much irrelevant information) into their developing minds. Enter Riemann and Speigelhalder and the interplay of REM sleep and SWS in this phenomenon. They suggest, from their own work and from reviewing the numerous studies published in this field over many years that, as we have seen, SWS is essential for the consolidation of memory, but also that REM sleep is critically important in the forgetting of irrelevancies (Landmann et al., 2014), please see Figure 4 below:

This novel set of studies leads us to our current understanding that SWS is necessary for (1) forming new schemas; and (2) incorporating new information into pre-existing schemas. Furthermore, that REM sleep is important for breaking-up schemas that are no longer of use to us. The implications of this are very significant for all mental health conditions; and we will look more into these in Chapter Five, but before we leave this section and look at age-related changes in sleep a final thought on REM sleep as important for schema disintegration. A connexion to something else that is new and exciting in psychology

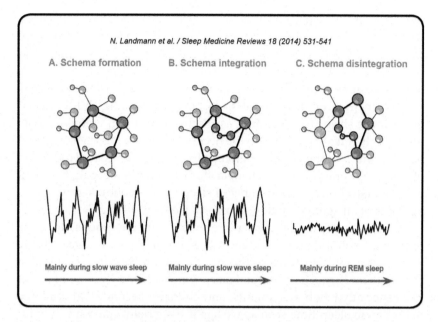

N. Landmann et al. / Sleep Medicine Reviews 18 (2014) 531-541

Figure 4. The memory and the forgettery, REM sleep and SWS.

in the twenty-first century, and that many healthcare professionals are now trained in the use of. Francine Shapiro's eye movement desensitization reprocessing (EMDR), whereby traumatic memories are treated (sometimes highly successfully and often with breathtaking speed) by focusing on the traumatic thought(s) and tracking the eyes left and right whilst holding the thought(s) in mind (Shapiro, Vogelmann-Sine, & Sine, 1994). Interestingly, this bilateral stimulation can also be emulated by touch and even sound alternating side-to-side. Perhaps then, we all do EMDR on ourselves, several times every night when we are sleeping, deconstructing unnecessary information during our multiple and frequent bouts of REM sleep? Perhaps too, here is an explanation as to the often highly emotional experiences of REM sleep dreams, that this emotional "venting" may be related to resolving trauma, much as EMDR does using bilateral stimulation whilst awake?

Age-related changes

We have probably all heard the old wives' tale that we need eight hours of sleep per night to feel well and function effectively during our waking lives. It is an interesting question to ask ourselves, and is certainly useful in the therapeutic situation with people who have insomnia, "how much sleep do I need?" Some people will want eight hours, but for others that can be hugely inappropriate, especially for infants and small children. Any parent will be acutely aware of the effects of tiredness on their children, and a small child will suffer enormously if they are only getting eight hours of sleep per night. Young children need much more sleep than this and, as discussed in the previous section, this is highly likely to be due to the necessity of sleep for schema formation, integration, and disintegration. Below in Figure 5 is a reproduction of a very old graph of sleep changes throughout the lifespan, based on a meta-analysis of a large number of sleep studies conducted with participants of all ages (Roffwarg, Muzio, & Dement, 1966).

Figure 5 shows a non-linear representation of age groups along the horizontal axis and hours of night-time sleep up the vertical axis. There are a few notable features of this graph that are worthy of attention. Firstly, there is much more total sleep time required by younger people, especially newborns, infants, and children. Second, that the large reduction in sleep time seen as we age is essentially complete by mid-adolescence, with total sleep time remaining fairly consistent from the

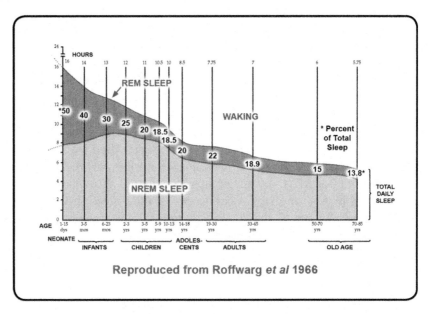

Figure 5. Sleep changes across the lifespan.

late teenage years right through until the end of our lives. Thirdly, that this reduction is mostly seen at the expense of losing REM sleep, with amounts of non-REM sleep remaining fairly constant throughout life (another reason why REM sleep was regarded as an optional extra for adults, but seemingly very important for children). We now have a pretty clear idea that this abundance of REM sleep in children is highly likely to be due to their need to disintegrate, or forget, lots of extraneous information allowing them to build useful and useable schemas for their developing minds. Finally, the numbers in the REM sleep area of the graph represent the percentage of the night's sleep that is occupied by REM sleep. Again this drops off radically throughout childhood as schemas develop and become set, but there is still a significant proportion of REM sleep that remains throughout our lives, as we all have a need to learn important information (in SWS), and so forget unimportant information (in REM). Sleep length then can vary depending on how old we are and this is a very useful point of departure in therapeutic terms when working with people who do not sleep well. With this in mind it is very important to note here that the curve on Figure 5 represents an *average* sleep time for people at various ages; an envelope above and below this line average line could be superimposed onto this curve to capture the sleep of both the long and short sleepers. It is important to note that people can be either short sleepers, sleep for an average amount of time, or be long sleepers for their age at *any* age, and most people (if they have capacity) will be able to tell you how much sleep they feel that they need and when they would like to take it. We will return to these ideas of sleep preference, chronotype (please see the next section of this Chapter) and short/long sleepers, later in this book on the treatment of insomnia in Chapters Five and Six, but it is also necessary to consider the type of person who we are, or whom we may find in our clinic.

Earlier in this chapter in section C. Sleep stages, we saw a simplified hypnogram from a healthy younger person when discussing the sleep stages, this is presented again below in Figure 6 immediately following this in Figure 7 is a similar simplified hypnogram for a typical "older" person, over the age of sixty-five years.

If we examine these two Figures (6 and 7) together there are some key changes to note in sleep as our age advances into older adulthood. First, the sleep of older people is lighter than that experienced by children and younger people. The Raphe nuclei and the pedunculopontine

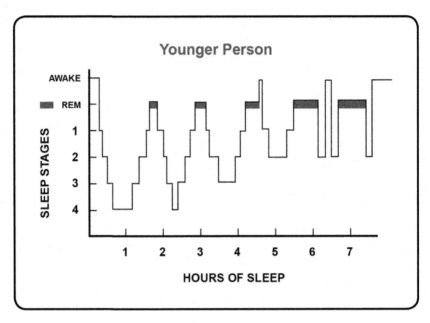

Figure 6. A simplified hypnogram from a typical younger person.

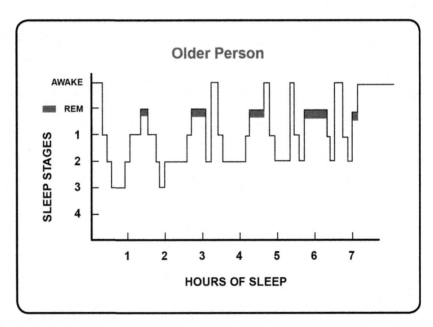

Figure 7. A simplified hypnogram from a typical older person.

areas of the brainstem are key areas that are crucial in the initiation and maintenance of sleep, and in the cycling of the sleep states (REM sleep and non-REM sleep) and shifts through the non-REM sleep stages one, two and three. The function of these areas depreciates as we age, so impacting negatively on the experience of sleep. Younger people with "fit" and resilient brains have Raphe nuclei and pedunculopontine areas which push people readily into their sleep, maintain it very effectively and control shifts thorough the sleep states and stages very well. Unfortunately, older people do not have such effective control and maintenance of their sleep as a result of these normal age-related changes to these regions of the brain. The upshot of this is that older people have sleep that is lighter and more easily disturbed than younger people. Figure 7, above, shows an absence of the deepest stage of non-REM sleep and a significant increase in night-time arousals when compared with the sleep of younger people, shown in Figure 6. A further complication for older people is that of similarly normal, age-related weakening of the sphincter muscles around the bladder and urethra, leading to an increased need to arise and void during the night. Unfortunately, these are normal, age-related changes that cannot be altered, and this is why older people complain more about their sleep than do the young (Bliwise, 1993).

Chronotypes

We have seen how our age impacts on our need for sleep, but then there is a question about when we sleep and certain people have certain preferences. There have, for a long time, been identified three chronotype subgroups, the first are people who like to rise early and get to bed early the so-called "morning larks", those at the other end of the spectrum, the "night owls" and the third group who are neither larks nor owls and have no particular preference, the intermediate type, or "ambivalents" (Horne & Ostberg, 1976). Some very recent work conducted in Russia has subdivided the ambivalent group into two further chronotypes. This research collected together around 140 healthy adults and sleep deprived them completely for twenty-four hours, and then assessed their performance (using reaction time testing) for the next twenty-four hours. They replicated previous research by finding that the group split fairly evenly into the three chronotypes, with around a third performing well in the morning, but not in the evening (the larks), a third performed well in the evening, but not in the morning (the owls), and a remaining third—the ambivalents. Their interesting finding came from further examination of the performance of the ambivalent group. This group were noticed to subdivide into two new chronotypes, the first were energetic and performed well across the twenty-four hours of testing and the second were lethargic and performed poorly throughout the twenty-four hours of testing all after a full day and night of sleep deprivation (Putilov, Donskaya, & Verevkin, 2015). The researchers did not go so far as to provide names for these two new chronotypes, but "swift" has been proposed for the energetic–ambivalent group and, unfortunately, "dodo" for the lethargic–ambivalent subgroup. Again, as with sleep length, the timing of sleep is also important for us and useful to ask about in therapy. A case example:

> Terry is in his mid-seventies and has been diagnosed with Alzheimer's disease for four years. His dementia has progressed to the point where he is often confused and has difficulty communicating. He has been an inpatient in an older adult mental health ward for the last six months as his wife had been unable to continue caring for him at home. Terry has always been a night owl, regularly rising at around 10am and rarely going to bed before 1am, but, since being on the ward, he has had difficulty adjusting to the routine of the ward, where patients are woken at 7am and given breakfast at 8am, and where they are encouraged to go to bed at 9pm as night staff come onto the ward at 10pm. Terry was often agitated and upset about being woken early in the morning and being put into his bed early in the evening and has been seen to exhibit "challenging behaviour". As a result he has been prescribed with sedative and antipsychotic medications. This has had a profoundly negative impact on his quality of life and exacerbated his rate of cognitive decline.

This is a common story for many people like Terry in hospital and residential care environments around the developed world today. The question remains: would Terry have been happier if he (or his wife if he was having trouble communicating) had been asked about his twenty-four-hour routine; and, even if he was asked, would this have made any difference to the routine of the ward on which he was living?

We are getting better at delivering "person centred care" and we are collecting personal biographies about the likes and dislikes of older people as they become institutionalised in order to tailor care programmes for them. But there is still some distance to travel, and these questions about sleep preferences are fundamental ones that are often overlooked and often lead to potentially unnecessary pharmacological "solutions" for Terry and many, many people like him.

Chronotypes are worthy of examination, and each of us will instinctively know how much sleep we need and when we like to get it. We will again revisit chronotypes in the assessment and treatment chapters of this book. Next though we return to some fundamental physiology of sleep and examine the impact that exposure to light, especially daylight, has on our sleep.

The influence of light

Many of us will remember being on the beach as children, or playing outside all day, and hearing our mothers or fathers saying something like: "he/she will sleep well tonight with all that fresh air". Well it is not the fresh air, it is the exposure to bright, natural light, and the effect that this has on our brains to produce the hormone and neurotransmitter melatonin, that is having the positive effect on our sleep.

There are specific receptors in our eyes which transmit their signals directly through the optic nerve to the suprachiasmatic nucleus (SCN) in the hypothalamus. This direct transmission of light from the retinas of our eyes aids the SCN in adjusting to "daytime", which is why our circadian rhythms can reset, or adjust, to a changing day length and time, for example, seasonal changes, autumnal and spring clock changes, jet lag and shift work (Moore-Ede, Sulzman, & Fuller, 1982). Visual transmissions from the eyes continue onward down the optic nerves to where the information is processed in the back of our brains, in the occipital region, but it is the direct transmission to the hypothalamus, the SCN and then on to the pineal gland that interests us here.

The pineal gland is a small organ within the brain, just behind the hypothalamus, the shape of a small pine cone, hence "pineal". The function of the pineal gland is to produce the hormone and neurotransmitter melatonin. The more light (and the more powerful the light) that hits our eyes, the greater the signal transmitted through the optic nerves to the hypothalamus, the SCN, and on to the pineal gland. As we have seen, the hypothalamus and SCN use this information to recognise that it is daytime and this aids in the entrainment of the circadian rhythm to the twenty-four-hour routine of life. The pineal gland though is stimulated by this "light pressure" and produces melatonin. The more light pressure it receives; the more melatonin it produces. Then, when the signal stops, that is, when the sun goes down, it gets dark, and there is no more light pressure, the pineal gland then releases its load of melatonin out into the brain and blood stream. This flood of melatonin helps to tell us that it is time to sleep, and it also has mild sedative properties, although its major potency is as a circadian rhythm regulator, which aids in telling our brains that it is time for sleep (Arendt, 2000).

Sound pressure is measured in decibels, but light pressure uses the units of "lux". Typical house lighting ranges from around 50 lux–300 lux, brighter office environments range from around 500 lux–800 lux, which is still much less than the light pressure that we receive from natural daylight. Even on a very overcast day we still receive around 1,000 lux from the sun through the clouds. A particularly clear and bright day can provide us with around 10,000 lux–25,000 lux, and direct sunlight perhaps up to 50,000 lux. We saw earlier in this section how light, and more accurately, light pressure, impacts on our eyes, retinas, optic nerves, hypothalamus, and pineal gland to influence the production of melatonin. Now we can see from the huge increase in light pressure that we receive in the outdoors how the beneficial effects of a day on the beach influences our sleep.

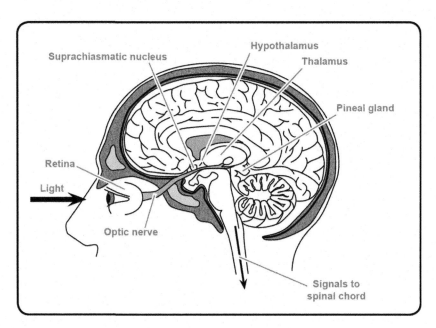

Figure 8. The effect of light on our brains.

Figure 8 on the previous page shows how light, after hitting our retinas, stimulates our optic nerve and passes signals into the deeper control centres of our brains (notably the hypothalamus, the SCN and the pineal gland).

This section has explored the influence of light on our sleep, which is a perhaps less well acknowledged phenomenon that impacts on sleep. The next section however, deals with the most well-known influence on our sleep, tiredness.

The sleep homeostat

The pressure that we feel to sleep is directly proportional to the amount of time that we have spent awake. If you have just had a normal amount of sleep for your system and have been awake for long enough to fully wake-up (maybe thirty minutes or so after getting up), and are then asked to get back into bed and go to sleep, getting to sleep again will be very difficult for you. You will have just spent the preceding six to nine(ish) hours relieving your sleep pressure (resetting your sleep homeostat to zero), and so will have little or no sleep pressure, or tiredness. Assuming of course that this preceding sleep was of good quality and that you have woken refreshed. If, however, you have just been awake for forty-eight hours, perhaps on a series of flights to travel to the other side of the world, and with no opportunities for sleep on the trip, then your sleep homeostat will be sky-high, you will be very, very tired, and you will find it very easy to initiate sleep. Below in Figure 9 is perhaps the simplest graph that you will ever see, providing an illustration of the effect of wakefulness and sleep on our pressure to sleep, also referred to as the homeostatic sleep drive.

As we can see in Figure 9, the longer that we remain awake, the greater our pressure to sleep, or tiredness will be. Every twenty-four hours we relieve this pressure by sleeping and our tiredness diminishes (inside the grey box on Figure 9). Then, once we have attained the necessary sleep for our systems, the sleep homeostat is reset and we awaken, refreshed, and without any pressure to sleep, until we have been awake for another full and active day. Should we not sleep then our tiredness will continue to increase as the homeostat is not being reset by sleep (the dotted line on Figure 9). This is of course very obvious, and we all know the feelings of tiredness associated with long periods of wakefulness, we will return to the sleep homeostat at the end of this chapter. Before then though, there are just a few more

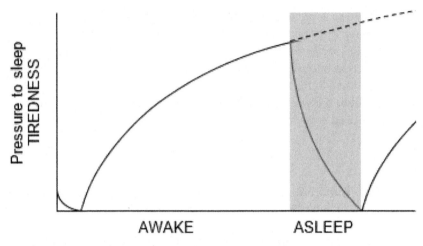

Figure 9. The homeostatic sleep drive.

things to consider in terms of sociological, physiological, and psychological impacts on our sleep.

Time givers

Our sleep and circadian rhythm is also influenced by "social time". If we are placed in a situation where we receive no social time-cues, for example, if we are placed into an environment without any clocks, sunshine, or other indicators to what the time of day (or night) is, then our circadian rhythm begins to free-run, and we adapt to a different day length driven by our suprachiasmatic nucleus (SCN). Our SCN is entrained to a twenty-four-hour day by external time cues, also referred to as *"zeit-gebers"* from the German: *"zeit"* meaning "time", and *"geber"* meaning "giver". The evidence for this came from a classic study conducted on himself by Michel Siffre in 1962 in France. Siffre took himself off to a deep cave without any external time cues of any kind (sunlight, clocks, communication with the outside world etc.) for around two months. He found that his circadian rhythm began to "free-run" and extended to a time beyond twenty-four hours (around twenty-five hours in his case). This initial study has been replicated under different conditions with larger numbers of participants many times and by many different research groups across the world. Probably the most influential set of studies were conducted by in the 1970's and 1980's.

These studies involved taking groups of people and placing them into "time-free" environments and have demonstrated a number of important findings. First, that a de-synchrony of the circadian rhythm from the twenty-four-hour day occurs with individuals experiencing desynchronised circadian rhythms in the range of around twenty-three to twenty-five hours when placed into time-free environments for long periods. Second, that the body temperature rhythm and the circadian rhythm of sleep and wakefulness, which are usually entrained and promote shifts to and from wakefulness and sleep, become decoupled. To give an example of this: you may well be familiar with feeling cold when tired at, or around, your usual bedtime. This is because your circadian rhythm of alertness is dipping in tandem with a dip in your circadian rhythm of body temperature (when occurring concurrently these dips are sleep-promoting). Conversely, in the morning, you may sometimes feel hot in bed in the mornings as your circadian rhythm of alertness is reaching a peak in tandem with a peak in body temperature (again, when occurring concurrently, such peaks are wakefulness-promoting). Finally, these studies collectively demonstrate the importance of external time-cues, or zeitgebers, (particularly light) in entraining the circadian rhythm to a twenty-four-hour day (Aschoff et al., 1971; Czeisler et al., 1999; Djik, Duffy, & Czeisler, 2000). We need these social cues to regulate our circadian rhythms, and, when they are altered, we experience negative effects to our functionality as a direct result of a desynchronisation of our circadian rhythms. Two very well recognised examples of alterations to our circadian rhythms by changing zeitgebers are shift work and jet lag. We will return to these two phenomena in the next section on the physiological impacts of sleep.

Physiological impacts

Sleep is a physiological process that is driven by a collection of electrical and chemical processes that occur, without our awareness, in our brains every twenty-four hours (usually). But that is not the whole story, our psychology—how we think and feel, also has a significant impact on how we sleep, and how we feel about it. The psychological impact on our sleep we will examine in the next section and further in Chapters Five and Six, but here we will explore some of the physiological impacts that there are on our sleep. The first, and perhaps most influential is the circadian rhythm. We looked at this in detail in previous sections of this chapter, but, as alluded to earlier, two phenomena implicate the particular significance of the circadian rhythm on our sleep, those of jet lag and shift work. There has been much research into the impact of these two phenomena on our sleep and performance. The shift work studies are of interest, especially those studies which have compared mortality and morbidity in people whom have worked shifts for many years, in comparison to those who have consistently worked more normal, or "social" hours. The now classic "nurse" studies are of particular interest and indicate the importance of the circadian rhythm on our long-term health.

Nurses are a useful population to study in this respect as many nurses work shifts while others work more conventional "nine–five" hours, providing two useful, "natural" populations to study whom are very similar in all other respects. When controlling for things like gender, age, income-level, years of education, socio-economic status, other illnesses etc. we see that shift-working nurses have a much increased rate of morbidity (illness) and mortality (they tend to die at a younger age) than those colleagues who have worked more conventional hours during their nursing careers. The extent to which morbidity and mortality rates increase in the shift-working groups is dependent on a few factors: (1) the number of years the shift-working has been going on for; (2) the frequency of rotation of the shifts; and (3) the more unsocial the hours. So people who have been working shifts, which rotate rapidly, shift from night to day shifts and whom have been doing this for many years will be the most at risk of increased morbidity and mortality. These findings indicate the importance of a regular circadian rhythm on our health and wellbeing long-term. Persistently shifting one's circadian rhythm has long-term detrimental effects on our physical health. The exact mechanisms by which our physical health deteriorates under conditions of circadian rhythm shifting and inadequate sleep are complex, they are still very much under investigation, and it is beyond the remit of this book to enter into a lengthy exploration of this broad area. Suffice it to say, the so-called "stress" hormone cortisol has a fundamental impact on our physical health, and this is raised under conditions of sleep deprivation and circadian rhythm disruption. Furthermore, the hormone melatonin is depleted under conditions of sleep deprivation and circadian rhythm disturbance; and this has a known influence on the development of some cancers, especially breast and colorectal cancers (Davis, Mirick, & Stevens, 2001; Schernhammer et al., 2003).

Jet lag has long been known to have more short-term negative impacts, particularly on our performance, with pilots and associated air staff legally required to have regular stopover breaks, especially on long haul routes, to enable them to rest appropriately before flying again. Similarly, there is legislation for long-distance lorry drivers to take breaks in their driving regularly every few hours and to rest for appropriate lengths of time in every twenty-four-hour period of work, in order to maintain safety in their driving occupations.

Focusing more specifically on sleep deprivation, as opposed to circadian rhythm disruption that occurs in shift workers and people under conditions of jet lag, there are a few more physiological impacts that are worthy of mention. We have seen above that blood pressure, the incidence of some cancers and cortisol levels are raised under conditions of sleep deprivation and circadian rhythm disturbances. However, we also now know that there is a significant link between sleep deprivation (both partial and total) and the development of Type 2 diabetes, obesity, and cardiovascular disease (Nedeltcheva & Scheer, 2014). The development of these conditions has implicated inefficient glucose metabolism and insulin production with respect to Type 2 diabetes (Donga et al., 2010), and the hormones leptin (reduced) and ghrelin (increased) with regard to obesity. Interestingly studies have found that partial sleep restriction impacts negatively on the balance of these hormones in both adults and children (Aldabal & Bahammam, 2011). These findings have stark implications for a twenty-four/seven society, whereby many people are "optionally" sleeping less in order to maintain busy professional and social lives at the expense of getting enough, good quality sleep.

There are a few other conditions which have a physiological impact on our sleep which we will return to in Chapter Four when we will look at the impact of some types of medication on our sleep, and again in Chapter Six where we will examine the impact on sleep in people with more complex presentations. The next section however will explore some of the psychological impacts on our sleep which have important ramifications for the treatment of sleep problems and insomnia.

Psychological impacts

How we think and feel not only affects our waking lives, but also has a significant impact on our sleep, especially our ability to initiate and maintain the sleeping states. There has long been an established link between a large number of "mental health" conditions and poor sleep. In fact, one would be hard pressed to find anyone living with an enduring mental health condition who does not have a concomitant sleep problem. Mental health conditions and insomnia almost universally seem to come hand-in-hand, with insomnia being a core diagnostic feature of many mental health conditions (e.g., major unipolar depression, bipolar depression, Lewy Body Dementia and so on). We also have good evidence for effective co-treatment (particularly for depression with co-morbid insomnia) (Manber et al., 2008), and emerging evidence for the co-treatment for other conditions, for example, people living with chronic pain and co-morbid insomnia (Tang, 2009), but we will return to these later after a brief examination of the interactive nature of sleep and our "mental" health.

There is an emerging school of thought that a large number of mental health conditions (notably those which tend to be acquired (e.g., depression and anxiety) rather than those to which people are more genetically predisposed (e.g., schizophrenia)) are regarded as disorders of memory. To expand and taking depression as an example of this: we know that people with depression are prone to certain thought processes that are involved in the development and maintenance of the condition. These are referred to as "cognitive bias" and "selective attention". Depressed people will tend to focus on negative situations or stimuli more than on more positive or neutral situations or stimuli (selective attention), and they will tend to see situations as more desperate than people who do not suffer from depressive symptomatology (cognitive bias). These two phenomena interact and, over time, can contribute to the maintenance and increasing severity of a depressive episode; and so lead an individual into a persistently and deeply depressed state of mind—major, clinical, unipolar depression. This process is almost always accompanied by poor sleep and, as mentioned above, insomnia is a core diagnostic feature of major depression.

If we reflect briefly on the section above on memory and schemas where we introduced the analogy of the sleeping brain being a cluttered office which is being "tidied" of superfluous information. If our sleep is disturbed then this "clutter" is not being fully cleared away before we awaken in the morning, leaving us feeling discombobulated with an "untidy" office still in need of some spring cleaning. If we look at this in terms of slow wave sleep and REM sleep on the formation, integration, and disintegration of schemas as proposed by Reimann's group in 2014, then this idea carries some weight. In that, if we do not get enough good quality sleep to arrange our memories effectively during the night, then the consequences of this are potentially twofold. First, our schemas are not as well organised as they could be, and this "cluttering" potentially aids in the precipitation and maintenance of a depressed mood; and second, that we begin to build new schemas for selective attention and cognitive bias (to negative situations or stimuli) and so the depressive state becomes self-perpetuating, even hard-wired into our neural pathways.

This idea is relatively novel, requiring further research to explore in detail and also explored for other mental health conditions, but the principle remains sound and extends beyond depression and into other mental health conditions. For example, people with depression (as above) will be developing schemas that selectively attend, and are more cognitively and emotionally biased towards, negative, threatening situations and events, which contributes further to their depression and to strengthening these schemas. Depressed people tend to regard the world as a depressing place. The same is true for people with anxiety—situations and events are perceived as worrisome, events that others (in health) might regard as trivial, are regarded as threatening or dangerous in some way. People with insomnia regard the bed as a place of arousal and distress rather than solitude and rest, and they attend to sleep-related stimuli more than people who sleep well (Speigelhalder, Espie, Nissen, & Riemann, 2008). Those whom have a dependency on alcohol, or eating, or gambling etc. will have schemas that selectively attend to the environment and see opportunities to drink, eat, gamble etc. more so than those who are less dependent. They have schemas that attune themselves towards these particular stimuli.

The argument here is that over time we become hard-wired (neurones become laid down and organised in our brains) to selectively attend to, and to have emotional and cognitive biases towards, certain situations or stimuli. There are three old adages here that can perhaps contextualise this as part of a brief thought experiment: One: "everyone has their drug", two "moderation in all things", and three "we see the world through rose-tinted spectacles". By way of example: A small amount of alcohol consumption is not regarded as harmful, it is even seen as protective of health by some. Conversely, excessive amounts of exercise can be harmful (and are part of the diagnostic criteria for some of the eating disorders), but we are often told that alcohol is a bad thing and that exercise is good for us. If we are using alcohol, or exercise, (or whatever) to excess then we may be "over-attending" to such an activity, and that leads to strengthened schemas for (and a cognitive bias towards) such activities and if these then start to predominate in our lives, then we may begin to "lose balance" and our mental health can begin to suffer as a result.

So if mental health conditions can be seen as a disorder of memory, and if memory is schematically organised, driven, and arranged; then sleep, which has such a pivotal role in that schematic organisation and arrangement, must be regarded as fundamental to the maintenance of our mental health, whether that be healthy or poorly, and everywhere else in between.

Pulling it all together

The previous sections have explored various aspects of sleep from a number of different vantage points. The view of sleep as an "off" state where not much happens has hopefully been fully dispelled, and some ideas about how important good quality sleep is to us hopefully has been made more apparent. The picture is complex, with the last thirty or so pages providing a brief summary of the various and most salient aspects of what, and how, it is to sleep, as far as our collective knowledge currently stands. Perhaps the best way to summarise this chapter and capture the complexity of the subject is with a visual representation of the factors that can influence our sleep. This representation is portrayed below in Figure 10. The figure is organised in an attempt to separate out the different components which mediate, moderate, and control our sleep and we will return to various elements of this figure time and again in further chapters of this book, particularly in relation to the assessment (Chapter Three) and treatment (Chapters Four and Five) of insomnia and the sleep of vulnerable groups (Chapter Six).

Figure 10 below is organised with different elements grouped together in terms of their collective function in an effort to simplify the complex mechanisms that can influence our sleep. Oval shapes indicate the collective influence and interactions of the circadian rhythm, the pineal gland, melatonin, and the influence of light and dark on our sleep. The homeostatic sleep drive element is shown with a hexagon. Social time is shown within a circle, age within a square, and how we think and feel, the last element covered in the previous section of this

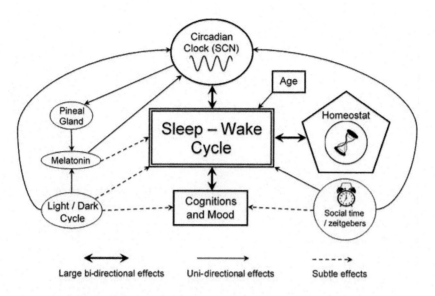

Figure 10. The mediating, moderating, and control factors of sleep.

chapter, within a rectangle. Some of these elements have a large impact on our sleep (and sleep has a large impact on them) and these relationships are shown with large bi-directional arrows (e.g., cognitions and mood), other elements have more singular, unidirectional effects (e.g., age), whilst others have subtler effects (e.g., zeitgebers on our mood). Some of the influences on our sleep are physiological (e.g., light), some are psychological (e.g., mood), and others are sociological (e.g., social time). This figure is a useful point of departure in terms of how to assess a sleep problem (i.e., using it as a template to examine where problems may be arising from) and where one direct attention for the successful treatment of a problem with sleep (and where one can intervene as a therapist) and we will return to this in Chapters Four and Five. However, before turning our attention to the assessment and treatment of insomnia we first need a definition, which will begin the next chapter on insomnia and the parasomnias.

CHAPTER TWO

Insomnias and the parasomnias

The previous chapter examined the "science of sleep" in relation to the various physiological, psychological, and sociological influences on sleep. This examination culminated in Figure 10 which summarised the complexity of what, and how, it is to sleep; showing the various controlling, moderating, and mediating factors that can influence our sleep. We will return to many of these elements in further chapters of this book, but before that a description of the various types of insomnia and how we assess sleep problems is warranted. This is crucial from the perspective of the therapist: a good formulation is essential for an effective treatment.

A definition of insomnia

There are various bodies and institutions around the world whom define diagnostic criteria for the whole gamut of human conditions, both physical and psychological. Insomnia is variously defined by many of these bodies and institutions (e.g., the World Health Organization, The ICD–10 (*the International Statistical Classification of Diseases and Related Health Problems*), DSM-V (the *Diagnostic and Statistical Manual of Mental Disorders*), and the *International*

Classification of Sleep Disorders published by the American Academy of Sleep Medicine). Although there is some variation on the exact definitions of the insomnias, there is broad agreement on the key criteria for these conditions which we will examine below. Insomnia is a significant problem with four–twenty-two per cent of the general population (proportions depending on the exact criteria used) reporting significant problems with sleep, proportions that increase with advancing age (Roth et al., 2011) and precipitate huge costs to society (Sivertsen & Nordhus, 2007). For the remainder of this chapter and book we will refer to the DSM-V criteria, as these are the most recently updated at the time of writing, and tend to be the criteria most commonly referred to and so potentially the most useful from a therapeutic perspective.

* * *

Insomnia is broadly defined as a problem with either: the initiation; or maintenance of sleep; or early morning awakening; or non-restorative sleep; which occurs for at least three nights per week; has been occurring for at least three months*; and causes significant psychological, occupational, or sociological dysfunction during the daytime (*Some criteria use one month instead of three). To expand on this and to breakdown the three key domains required for a diagnosis of insomnia:

- There must be a problem with one or more of the following: getting to sleep, staying asleep, waking too early in the morning, or not feeling refreshed.
- That this problem has some level of chronicity, that is, that it occurs regularly and has been occurring for a significant period of time.
- The problem with sleep causes a significant level of dysfunction during the daytime.

These broad criteria have been used for many years, but have recently been updated in May 2014 after the release of the new *Diagnostic and Statistical Manual of Mental Disorders* version five (DSM-V). Below in Table 1 is a facsimile of the DSM-V criteria and we can see the three domains, identified above, within these criteria with some interesting additional ones, which we will discuss later.

Table 1. DSM-V criteria for chronic insomnia.

A. The predominant complaint is dissatisfaction with sleep quantity or quality. In children or the elderly, the complaint may be made by a caregiver or family member.

B. Report of one or more of the following symptoms:

 1. Difficulty initiating sleep. In children, this may be manifested as difficulty initiating sleep without caregiver intervention.
 2. Difficulty maintaining sleep, characterised by frequent awakenings or problems returning to sleep after awakenings. In children this may be manifested as difficulty returning to sleep without caregiver intervention.
 3. Early morning awakening with inability to return to sleep.
 4. Non-restorative sleep.
 5. In children, prolonged resistance to going to bed and/or bedtime struggles.

C. The sleep complaint is accompanied by significant distress or impairment in daytime functioning as indicated by the report of at least one of the following:

 1. Fatigue or low energy.
 2. Cognitive impairment (e.g., attention, concentration, memory).
 3. Mood disturbance (e.g., irritability, dysphoria).
 4. Behavioural problems.
    (e.g., hyperactivity, impulsivity, aggression).
 5. Impaired occupational or academic functioning.
 6. Impaired interpersonal/social functioning.
 7. Negative impact on caregiver or family functioning (e.g., fatigue, sleepiness).

D. The sleep difficulty occurs at least three nights per week.

E. The sleep difficulty is present for at least three months.

F. The sleep difficulty occurs despite adequate opportunity for sleep.

For a diagnosis of insomnia, an individual is required to experience one or more symptoms in all of the lettered criteria (A–F) above.

From previous editions of the DSM these criteria have been broadened out to include: sensitivity to the reports of caregivers of children and older people (whom may lack capacity to provide accurate information about themselves); to acknowledge the impact of the sleep disturbance on others; and also to include provision of adequate opportunity for sleep (in the modern twenty-four/seven society). There is also an expansion of the daytime dysfunction domain, with the inclusion of additional elements of fatigue, low mood, cognitive detriments, and (focused more on children) behavioural and academic consequences. The familiar criteria of: problems with sleep initiation, maintenance or early waking; frequency and chronicity; and daytime dysfunction are still clearly embedded within these updated criteria, and they are particularly useful when formulating a treatment plan for patients, a subject to which we will return in Chapters Four and Five. So, we have a set of criteria for the diagnosis of insomnia, but the picture is complicated a little further by a different set of insomnia and parasomnia "types". These are presented in Table 2 below.

Types of insomnia and parasomnia

Table 2. Different types of insomnia and parasomnia.

- Difficulty Initiating Sleep
- Difficulty Maintaining Sleep
- Early Morning Awakening
- Transient insomnia
- Acute insomnia
- Chronic insomnia
- Psycho-physiological (primary) insomnia
- Co-morbid insomnia
- Adjustment insomnia
- Circadian/schedule insomnia
    - Delayed sleep phase syndrome
    - Advanced sleep phase syndrome
    - Shift work
    - Jet lag
- Hypersomnia
- Parasomnias
    - Those parasomnias common in children
        - Nightmares
        - Sleepwalking (somnambulism)
        - Somniloquy
        - Enuresis
    - Those parasomnias occurring at any age
        - Night terrors

(Continued)

Table 2. (Continued)

- Bruxism
- Sleep paralysis
- REM sleep behaviour disorder
- Periodic leg movements
- Restless legs syndrome
  - The more unusual parasomnias
    - Sexsomnia
    - Sleep homicide
    - Sleep-related eating disorder
    - Exploding head syndrome
- Sleep Apnoea
  - Obstructive
  - Central
  - Catathrenia
- Narcolepsy
- Sleep-state misperception

The above table identifies a subset of insomnia and parasomnia types which underlie a diagnosis and we will expand on these below.

Difficulty initiating sleep (DIS)

In healthy sleepers the initiation of sleep usually takes between ten and twenty minutes. This time taken to initiate sleep is referred to as Sleep Onset Latency (SOL). If someone is taking longer than twenty minutes to get to sleep then they may be diagnosed with DIS if this problem is occurring for three or more nights per week, has been occurring for three months or longer, and is causing significant daytime dysfunction in one or more domains. Conversely, if an individual is initiating their sleep very quickly, that is, has a sleep onset latency of less than five minutes then this is an indication that they are very tired (have lots of sleep pressure); and so they may not be getting the appropriate amount of sleep for their age and sleep type. Mary Carskadon and William Dement invented the Multiple Sleep Latency Test (MSLT) in 1982 to test the sleepiness of individuals. The MSLT has become widely used in a number of clinical and research applications and has become a gold-standard method for testing the sleepiness of an individual. The MSLT comprises of asking the individual under test to get into bed and to try and initiate sleep in a conducive environment (i.e., without noise and light distractions). Usually this test is administered between one-and-a-half to three hours after waking, and is repeated throughout the day at two-hour intervals. The time taken to initiate sleep is then recorded on each occasion. If sleep is not initiated within twenty minutes, then the MSLT is aborted until the next test, two-hours later. The polysomnogram (more on this in the next section of this chapter) is used to detect sleep onset and also to establish whether sleep is initiated in a "normal" way, that is, entering stages one and two of non-REM sleep, rather than in an aberrant fashion, that is, entering REM very quickly, which may be an indication narcolepsy (Carskadon & Dement, 1982).

Difficulty maintaining sleep (DMS)

In healthy adults there should be minimal intrusion into night-time sleep. Multiple awakenings are common and normal in infants and these gradually decrease during the first year of life. Healthy children are usually capable of sleeping through the night after the age of eight to twelve months. If a person is waking during the night and not being able to re-initiate their sleep within fifteen minutes then they may be diagnosed with DMS, again, if this problem is occurring for three or more nights per week, if this problem has been on-going for more than three months, and if there are detrimental daytime consequences (Morin, 2003).

Early morning awakening (EMA)

Waking early in the morning and not being able to re-initiate sleep is also a recognised form of insomnia, common in some people with depression and alcohol dependency syndrome (both of which we will return to in Chapter Six). If an individual is waking thirty or more minutes before their preferred wake time and if their total sleep time is less than six-and-a-half hours (and again experiencing the same issues with frequency, chronicity, and daytime dysfunction as with DIS and DMS above) then they may be diagnosed with EMA insomnia (Morin, 2003).

Transient insomnia

This is a rarely used term in behavioural sleep medicine and refers to a problem with sleep that occurs for less than a week, it is unusual for people to present with this condition as the sleep problem has either self-corrected or progressed into another form (acute or chronic insomnia) before an appointment is made and met with a treating professional. Many of us will experience periods of transient insomnia, multiple times throughout our lives, but these usually self-correct relatively quickly.

Acute insomnia

As we saw above there is some difference of opinion around what constitutes a period of acute insomnia, with some criteria stating that poor sleep for around one month is required for a diagnosis, whereas other criteria stating a three-month period. Whichever criteria we use, acute insomnia is often stress-related, and often self-corrects, as in the case of transient insomnia above. Usually, unless there is a specifically identifiable trigger that requires immediate treatment, "watchful-waiting" is usefully employed in order to see if this acute period on insomnia does indeed self-correct, or whether it progresses into a more prolonged period of chronic insomnia.

Chronic insomnia

Again, as we saw earlier in this chapter, chronic insomnia is a problem with either DIS, DMS, EMA, or non-restorative sleep which occurs three or more times per week, for a period or three or more months and causes significant daytime dysfunction in one or more domains, be they psychological, occupational, or sociological. Chronic insomnia, may result from multiple causes, sometimes physiological (e.g., pain), sometimes psychological (e.g., depression) and sometimes social/ relational (e.g., bereavement), or indeed, there may be multiple presentations with physical symptoms, affecting psychological patterns, that in turn may affect social interactions, which can all combine to effect a state of chronically disturbed sleep. Take for example an individual living with chronic pain. The physical symptoms have a direct impact on the individual's ability to be comfortable in bed and to initiate sleep. These continual sensations of pain cause the individual to feel quite depressed. The lack of mobility due to the pain, and the lack of motivation due to the depression that the individual is experiencing, makes it difficult for that person to get out of the house and interact with others. This impacts on their ability to get some exercise and exposure to bright light, and so these three factors (physical, psychological, and social/environmental/relational) all combine to effect poor sleep in that person. This has important implications for treatment and we will look again specifically at people living with chronic pain in Chapter Six. Needless-to-say, the example given above identifies the sometimes complex nature of a presentation of insomnia, and the skill required of a treating healthcare professional in identifying all the salient triggers that a person may be experiencing, or may have experienced in the past. There is a requirement of the healthcare professional to identify these triggers in order to make an effective and accurate formulation and so design an effective treatment plan for that person. Below, in the following sections we will expand on some more subtypes of insomnia that were identified in Table 2 earlier in this chapter, some of which may be transient, acute or chronic, and may cause DIS, DMS, or EMA.

Psycho-physiological (primary) insomnia

People with psycho-physiological insomnia (PPI), also referred to as primary insomnia, present solely with a sleep complaint and without any other comorbidities. This is a very common diagnosis of insomnia, but, with careful assessment, there is often an underlying comorbidity, either physiological, psychological, social/relational or a combination. Once detected, the underlying comorbidity is usually worth considering and treating at the same time as the primary presentation of insomnia, often with enhanced results than treating either condition in isolation. If there are no other (obvious or more elusive) underlying conditions which may have an impact on the client's sleep, then an individual presenting with poor sleep may be diagnosed with PPI. The treatment of which we will consider in the next chapter before which we will spend some time looking at other forms of insomnia.

Comorbid insomnia

As the name suggests, people with comorbid insomnia have a problem sleeping alongside some other condition, which can be physiological, psychological, social/relational (or combined) in nature. Historically, insomnia in this domain was referred to as "secondary insomnia" and the treatment pathway involved treating the comorbidity and ignoring the "secondary" insomnia as this would be expected to self-correct after the successful management of whatever the presenting comorbidity was. For example, people with depression often do not sleep well and their poor sleep might traditionally have been regarded as a secondary insomnia resulting from their low mood. Treatment of the mood disorder (depression) would naturally precipitate an improvement in sleep. There was some sense to this as often sleep problems would improve after the successful treatment of the comorbid presentation. However, we now know that for several conditions (particularly depression and pain), that regarding the sleep problem as "comorbid" rather than "secondary" and treating the sleep problem *concurrently* with treatment as usual for the comorbid presentation has improved outcomes for both the sleep problem *and* the comorbidity in terms of: (1) a faster recovery time; (2) reduced relapse rates; and (3) maintenance of treatment effects. As in the example above, treating depression alongside treatment of the sleeping problem has shown faster improvements in mood and sleep outcomes compared with treatment for each condition in isolation, and that these improvements are maintained and less likely to relapse (Manber et al., 2008). Thus providing a strong argument for the concurrent treatment of "co-morbid" insomnia, and our (now) rejection of the label "secondary" insomnia. We will return to many of the commonly experienced comorbidities in Chapter Six where we will explore some specific considerations in assessment and treatment of the more common comorbid insomnias.

Adjustment insomnia

Adjusting to changes in life circumstances can often precipitate stress responses and we all experience these at multiple times throughout our lives. For example, going to "big school" for the first time, becoming a teenager, being bullied, falling in and out of love, going to university, starting a job, getting married, becoming pregnant and having children, being made redundant, separating and getting divorced, moving home, managing finances, being bereaved, managing illness and deteriorating health, providing care, getting ill, going into hospital or becoming institutionalised, and dying; all precipitate stress in our lives and may well lead to an adjustment insomnia. Should the adjustment be short-lived and "successful" any adjustment insomnia is likely to be transient or acute, and so self-correct, with the successful assimilation of whatever is being adjusted to into our lives. Sometimes though, the adjustment may be prolonged and this may precipitate a longer term, more chronic insomnia. Exploring what has been (or is being) adjusted to can often help to provide a useful formulation for the development and implementation of an effective treatment plan for the person with this kind of insomnia. Broadly speaking there are three domains into which adjustment insomnia can fall, these may act in isolation or, more commonly, be overlaid with one another. These domains are social, environmental, and psychological and are perhaps best explained with a couple of examples.

Anyone who has had a child will know what adjustment insomnia is all too well, and the adjustment insomnia operates across all three domains. Socially, there is another person in the house, and one who needs feeding every couple of hours regardless of the time of day (or night!). Environmentally there is a Moses basket or cot in the bedroom and another person whom snuffles, coughs, gurgles etc. during the night, when once there was no such intrusion into the sleeping environment. There is also the psychological element in play as there is the joy of a new member of the family, but also the distress of being chronically sleep deprived; and the wondering: "Will he sleep well tonight?" "When will she start to sleep through the night?" "When will this teething stop?" and, "How long will this head cold last?" And so on.

Another example:

George was made redundant from his factory job of thirty years. The regular routines under which he was used to living were no longer present in his life (*social*), he no longer went to work and spent much longer at home (*environmental*), he no longer saw his peers on a regular basis and began to feel isolated (*social/psychological*), and he no longer felt like a useful, taxpaying member of society (*psychological*).

George therefore experienced multiple consequences from a singular event, and his adjustment insomnia was obviously influenced from several different, but interacting directions. These are all important considerations for the therapist working with him.

Adjustment insomnias are extremely commonly occurring sleep problems, affecting everyone at some stage or other in our lives, and they can also be quite complex in their presentation, with each individual being differentially affected as a result of life's experiences. Imagine two different George's from the last example. George One hated his job, did not socialise with his peers, but enjoyed golf. In his enforced retirement he spent much longer on the golf course, and significant amounts of money behind the bar at the club. The financial worries and his alcohol dependency caused him to present with his insomnia. George Two loved his job, his colleagues were the sum total of his social life outside of work, and he missed the routine and the feeling of inclusion and productivity that his job provided him, and these were the reasons for him to present with insomnia. Obviously these two Georges require entirely different approaches to therapy, and it is the skill of the individual therapist to tease these differences out for each client, and so to deliver effective, person-centred treatment.

Circadian/schedule insomnia

Chronologically influenced insomnias are experienced by anyone who has experienced jet lag or worked unsocial hours. Others may have had times in their lives when they have been required to be awake at periods of time that were not usual for them. Most people with such schedule problems overcome them by adaptation (e.g., jet lag) or making certain lifestyle choices (e.g., choosing not to work night shifts). However, in a few individuals, there is an intractable and inflexible chronotype, which means that they find it very difficult to maintain a functional life under "normal" working hours, these are the delayed and advanced sleep phase syndromes.

Delayed sleep phase syndrome

Individuals with DSPS (also known as delayed sleep phase disorder (DSPD), or delayed sleep phase type (DSPT)) have a delayed chronotype which means that they preferentially arise later in the morning, or even early in the afternoon and find it very difficult to get to bed (and to sleep) before midnight and into the early hours of the morning. Several studies around the world have identified around 0.13 per cent–0.17 per cent of the population experience severe DSPS to the extent that they are "disabled" in their ability to function properly at work (Schrader, Bovim, & Sand, 1993; Yazaki, Shirakawa, Okawa, & Takahashi, 1999). Many of these people force themselves to adapt to more conventional working hours and experience insomnia as a result. These individuals are often misdiagnosed with primary (PPI) insomnia. Others will self-select employment that is more nocturnal in nature, to suit their particular extreme "owl" chronotype. Whereas others will make adaptations to their daily lives, by scheduling naps for example, in order to overcome the tiredness, they experience as a result of going to bed late (naturally), but forcing themselves from bed earlier than they would choose, in order to get to work, and so shortening their required sleep time. Although this latter strategy often proves unsuccessful as fatigue, excessive daytime sleepiness, and headaches are often reported and precipitate problems with maintaining academic or occupational performance (Okawa & Uchiyama, 2007). There have been calls for employers to recognise extreme DSPS as a disability and to make allowances for employees living with the condition. Treatments include: careful sleep scheduling, light therapy in the daytime, dark therapy in the later evening, melatonin and modafinil prescriptions (Sack et al., 2007; Dodson & Zee, 2010).

Advanced sleep phase syndrome

In a very similar fashion to the above section of DSPS, but in the opposite direction we have ASPS (also known as advanced sleep phase disorder (ASPD) or advanced sleep phase type (ASPT)). ASPS is less common than DSPS and has a strong genetic link with many people living with ASPS having relatives with the same condition. The Period2 gene (PER2) has been linked to ASPS (Toh et al., 2001). Unlike people with DSPS, most people with ASPS do not complain of daytime sleepiness and do not experience the problems that people with DSPS do with managing their employment. People with ASPS mostly cite missing-out on evening activities as their main difficulty. Commonly, people with ASPS may be sleeping from around 19:30 and arising at about 04:30. Epidemiological data is not available to report the exact proportion of the population whom experience ASPS, but the numbers of people with ASPS is likely to be very small (Sack et al., 2007).

Shift work

Much more of a common influence on poor sleep, experienced by very many people, is that of the impact of shift work on sleep. We discussed the chronic impact of regularly rotating shift patterns in Chapter One of this book, in the section on the physiological impacts on sleep, with shift-working implicated in reduced quality of life, and with increased morbidity and mortality rates in shift-workers. These are exacerbated by the longer time spent working shifts, the rapidity with which those shifts rotate, and the more antisocial the hours worked (e.g., night shifts). Increased stress hormones (especially cortisol) are implicated in this increased morbidity and mortality and are most certainly driven by inadequate amounts of sleep and continually adjusting and readjusting the circadian rhythm. As we will see later in Chapters Four and Five on the treatment of sleep problems, a routine is an essential part of a healthy sleep (and wake) pattern. With a consistent routine the circadian rhythms of sleep/wakefulness (alertness) and body temperature become synchronised, or entrained to each other. Concurrent dips in body temperature and alertness culminate in a strong signal for the induction of sleep (in the late evening), and concurrent rises in body temperature and alertness culminate in a strong signal to wake (in the morning). Rotating shift patterns disrupt the synchrony between these two rhythms, making sleep less easy to induce and to maintain. As a result, people living with frequently rotating shift patterns are continually disrupting the synchrony of their circadian rhythms and their sleep suffers as a result. The consequences of this are manifold. Long-term there are clearly established negative health consequences (Costa, 1996), but in the short- and medium-terms there are feelings of fatigue, and so impaired performance, which leads to mental health problems (Lac & Chamoux, 2004), decreased productivity and an increased rate of work-related accidents (Rajaratnam & Arendt, 2001).

Many employers are behind the curve in respect to their shift-working employees. Allowing workers to choose their own shifts (so owls can work the later shifts and larks the earlier ones) would enable employees to feel as though they are valued and have some autonomy in how they work. Selecting permanent shifts would mean that workers can synchronise to one working pattern and so avoid continually disrupting their circadian rhythms (with concomitant advantages to mental and physical health in the short-, medium- and longer-terms), and, on the back of these positive outcomes, employers would have a happier, healthier, more productive (and less accident prone) workforce. There would be less time taken off work with stress-related illness and less litigation involved in resolving work-related accident cases and complaints of unfair treatment by workers. A win win situation. The multiple employers whom adopt rapidly rotating (often two-week rotation patterns) in order to maximise efficiency, and so productivity, in the short-term are almost certainly shooting themselves in the foot in the medium- and longer-terms, spending their short-term profits on sickness and litigation payouts later on.

Jet lag

Many of us will have experienced jet lag and, usually, this is not a problem for us, especially if we are heading out on a well-earned and much anticipated holiday in an exciting and exotic place. The anticipation and excitement can offset the negative consequences of jet lag. For some groups of people though, jet lag can be a particular problem. Notably pilots (and other airline staff) and business people who regularly fly around the world for work. These groups can find jet lag has a significant negative effect on them. The mechanisms by which jet lag affects people are exactly the same as for those described in the previous section on shift-workers, and are more of an issue for people whom travel regularly and for those whom travel through a greater number of time zones.

We all experience mild jet lag in the United Kingdom every autumn and spring when our clocks change backwards and forwards, respectively by one hour for daylight saving. This is a similar experience to travelling to a nearby country, where the time is adjusted by just one or two hours, the experience of jet lag is minimal, and adapted to very quickly. Considering long-haul flights, however, where one is transported through many time zones, then more of a negative impact is experienced. Anyone who has travelled to, say, Australia from the UK, or back the other way, and has experienced a complete day–night reversal will know these feelings well. Fatigue, tiredness, and sleep disturbances are the most obvious, but there are also subtler effects of nausea, hunger, and gastric upsets in some people. Usually adaptation to the new time zone is made within a couple of weeks (even after a complete day–night reversal) as a result of zeitgebers in the new time zone assisting in the resetting of our circadian rhythms. However, we often then return from our two-week holidays only to have to reset our circadian rhythms again, but this time without the anticipation and excitement of a holiday to look forward to, just the imminent return to work.

In humans the circadian rhythm tends to be slightly longer than twenty-four hours, and, as a result, the circadian rhythm tends to free-run naturally in a forwards (or phase delaying) direction (Czeisler, Zimmerman, Ronda, Moore-Ede, & Weitzman, 1980). This is why people generally find it easier to stay up later and sleep in later than usual, rather than to go to bed earlier and get up earlier than usual. With respect to jet lag, this is why westerly travel (where the time zones phase delay with the circadian rhythm) has less of an impact on us than easterly travel, where time zones are phase advancing.

Hypersomnia

As we saw in the Chapter One there are certain sleep types, or chrono-types, the short, medium (normal length), and long sleepers, and the larks, the owls, and the "ambivalents" (the swifts and the dodos). The vast majority of the adult human population will sleep from between six and nine hours in every twenty-four-hour period and every human adult whom has capacity will be able to tell you how much sleep they would like, and when they would like to get it. There is one form of insomnia in the list described above in Table 2 that is not related to a lack of sleep, rather an excess of it, that of hypersomnia. Bizarrely the symptoms of over-sleeping are much the same as for not sleeping enough. One would intuitively imagine that an excess of sleep should endow an individual with extra resources, increased feelings of energy, and added enthusiasm for life, but this is not the case. There are certain conditions and situations where an excess of sleep is required, but, as a general rule, over-sleeping provides a person with very similar symptoms to those experienced by the person with insomnia.

Rebound, or recovery, sleeping is becoming increasingly common in modern-day twenty-four/seven societies, with many individuals building up a sleep debt during a busy working-week, and then sleeping excessively at the weekends to recover. This is an all too common practice and is not a sustainable one in the long-term. The effects of such a boom-and-bust existence are likely to precipitate (in the long-term) the same symptoms as chronic shift work as described above. More immediately though, people engaging in such a lifestyle are likely to experience detriments to their performance and wellbeing during times of bust and, with a continually shifting routine, make themselves more vulnerable to the precipitation of a longstanding sleep problem. More on this later in this chapter when we will examine precipitating and perpetuating factors in the development and maintenance of insomnia.

In Chapter Six we will look in more depth at certain conditions that have an impact on sleep, however there are a few conditions which are noteworthy because of their relationship with over-sleeping that are worthy on mention here.

First, people whom are recovering from a stroke or a traumatic brain injury will often sleep for longer periods of time, especially in the immediate aftermath of the index incident and sometimes for several months afterwards, depending on the severity of the injuries to their brain. They are also prone to other sleep and wake disorders including parasomnias, fatigue/excessive daytime sleepiness, insomnia, sleep-disordered breathing, depression, and anxiety (Bassetti, 2005). It is important to consider the length of time since the injury and the severity of it in relation to estimating the amount of sleep such a person might be requiring. The "two-year" rule is often employed in traumatic brain injury cases, whereby two years after the index incident are required to have passed before the individual is considered to have had sufficient time for their brain to heal from their accident, to the fullest extent that it is likely to (Ruttan, Martin, Liu, Colella, & Green, 2008; Schretlen & Shapiro, 2003). There may often be a requirement for people in this period to require more sleep as part of the natural brain-healing process. Obviously this is a very loose rule-of-thumb and is very much dependent on the severity of the sustained injuries.

Second, there are a few other groups who also may be experiencing symptoms of hypersomnia and these can be notoriously difficult to treat, often as is it uncertain whether the amount of sleep taken is actually the amount of sleep that is required, and these are some people living with chronic pain (particularly fibromyalgia), Multiple Sclerosis (MS), Chronic Fatigue Syndrome (CFS) and Myalgic Encephalitis (ME). The very nature of these often highly disabling conditions frequently reduces mobility and enhances fatigue, and often people with these conditions find themselves resting, and at times, falling asleep as a result of reduced mobility and elevated fatigue. They will often sleep numerous times during the day and night, may not be getting their sleep in bed all the time, and often complain about feelings of fatigue and tiredness being a major barrier to their wellbeing. Good sleep practices, not over sleeping, sleeping in the bedroom, pacing of activities, and scheduling rest periods have all shown good results with this type of client (Bested & Marshall, 2015) and we will return to the various treatment strategies for sleeping problems in these groups of clients in Chapter Six.

Parasomnias

There are a number of conditions which occur in and around sleep that are a potential source of distress for many people, some are transient, some are developmental, others may be more familial or genetic in nature and yet others are of unknown origin and remain enigmatic in their presentations. There is an excellent book written on the more extreme, extravagant, and outrageous parasomnias, by Dr. Carlos Shenck called *Paradox Lost—Midnight in the Battleground of Sleep and Dreams—Violent Moving Nightmares, REM Sleep Behavior Disorder* (Schenck, 2005) for those interested in sleep homicide (see later in this chapter) and superhuman feats of strength and agility in sleep etc. Suffice it to say that it is not the remit of this book to explore all the weird and wonderful parasomnia presentations, but in the next few sections we will examine those that are more commonly seen in the treatment room. All the parasomnias listed below will all tend to manifest and/ or be more extreme in their presentation during times of stress, and this stress can be naturally occurring (e.g., by being excessively tired), or self-induced (e.g., by drinking alcohol or consuming some recreational, prescribed or over-the-counter drugs), or be situationally driven (e.g., bereavement, redundancy or separation).

Parasomnias can occur at any age, but there are certain ones that are more common in childhood, e.g., nightmares, sleepwalking, and enuresis (bedwetting), and we shall look at these first before considering those which can also occur at any age, namely: night terrors, bruxism (teeth grinding), sleep paralysis, periodic limb movements, and restless legs syndrome. This section on the parasomnias will then conclude with a brief examination of the more unusual parasomnias of sleep homicide, sexsomnia, exploding head syndrome, and sleep eating.

Those parasomnias common in children

Nightmares

Upsetting sleep imagery is a common occurrence in children (Bruni & Novelli, 2010), especially after the age of around three years old and often occurring as a result of daytime distress. Nightmares are very commonly seen in children who have experienced abuse or trauma, those of parents who are in a dysfunctional relationship, when moving house, being bullied at school, when anxious about examinations or sporting events, and also at transitions from junior, to middle, to senior schools as they adapt and settle into their new surroundings. If the nightmares are infrequent (less than a couple of nights per week) and are linked to a transient life experience (like changing school, for example) then they will usually abate and disappear in a relatively short space of time. If, however, the distress is more severe and prolonged then the nightmares may be more frequent and intense, and so require further intervention. The most effective psychobehavioural treatment for nightmares, that of imagery rehearsal, is described in detail in Chapter Four in Section B titled Imagery rehearsal.

Sleepwalking (somnambulism)

Again, bouts of sleepwalking can occur at any age, and are often (but not always) linked with upsetting dreams. Usually they are more prevalent under times of distress, as with nightmares above, and can be dangerous if people are leaving the house, or even climbing out of windows (defenestrating) in their sleep. A recent Italian report suggests that sleepwalking is regularly experienced by fifteen per cent of children (Bruni & Novelli, 2010).

Somniloquy

Somniloquy, also known as sleep talking, is also common in children, although it can occur at any age. Talking in sleep can range from inaudible mumbling, to clear, loud shouting and can occur in isolation, or co-present with another parasomnia, e.g., Sleepwalking, night terrors, or sleep-related eating disorder.

Enuresis

Bedwetting occurs in all children at some stage or other in their development, usually at around the time when they stop wearing nappies through the night. Some children will be dry through the night at quite a young age, with others taking some time to achieve consistently dry nights. There seems to be little to predict at what age a child will achieve consistently dry nights, although particularly deeply sleeping children may be more likely to wet the bed for longer than children who are lighter sleepers, as they are less likely to arise and use the bathroom during the night-time. This is a normal and natural developmental process in all children, however, children can also start to wet the bed when they are distressed in their daily lives and this may also be linked to their having nightmares. Bedwetting is exacerbated by feelings of shame and it is important for parents and carers to manage this without making the child feel guilty or ashamed about wetting the bed. A recent review suggests that around fifteen per cent of five year olds regularly experience nocturnal enuresis and that this is more common in boys than girls (DiBianco, Morley, & Al-Omar, 2014).

Although there is much evidence for the psychobehavioural management of the insomnias in children, much less research is available to advocate these for the use of childhood parasomnias. However, initial research in the area is beginning to emerge and demonstrate some good levels of effectiveness for these methods (Sadeh, 2005).

Those parasomnias occurring at any age

Night terrors

Night terrors are a relatively rare phenomenon affecting only a very few people. Many people think that they might be experiencing night terrors, but this is often a misdiagnosis of the much more commonly occurring nightmares. The distinction is relatively easy to make. Nightmares probably occur in all stages of sleep, but the ones that are remembered are occurring in stage two non-REM sleep or in REM sleep when the brain is relatively active and the person wakes from these states remembering their bad dream. Sleep terrors originate directly from stage three, deep, slow wave sleep, they are also characterised by (sometimes) blood curdling screams and extreme agitation, which can be quite distressing for anyone witnessing such an event. As a result of these very abrupt awakenings from deep sleep, people who have night terrors usually re-initiate their sleep quite quickly and have no memory of any negative dream imagery, either if woken fully at the time, or the next morning. They will often disbelieve their parent, carer or partner if they are told that they have had a bad dream, and may even resent them for waking them up to see if they are alright. Those experiencing nightmares, on the other hand, will often take some time to re-initiate their sleep (as they have awoken from a lighter stage of sleep and so will be at or near a peak in their circadian rhythm), they will also usually be able to recount what they have been dreaming about (at the time and also sometimes the following morning), whereas there is no memory of any distress following a night terror (Haupt, Sheldon, & Loghmanee, 2013). The management of sleep terrors in children has often utilised to prescription of medications (including melatonin) and, as there has been much evidence to support the use of psychobehavioural methods in the management of childhood insomnia, the use of these methods has been proposed for managing childhood parasomnias, with some initial research showing promise in this area (Sadeh, 2005).

Bruxism

Teeth grinding during sleep is another recognised parasomnia, that again can occur at any age. In extreme cases people are provided with moulded rubber mouthguards to wear during the night in order to prevent people experiencing this condition from grinding their teeth away. Extreme teeth grinding at night is relatively rare, but milder cases are common, and are exacerbated by similar triggers to all the parasomnias, i.e., daytime distress, over-tiredness, alcohol, and some medications (both prescribed and recreational) (Murali, Rangarajan, & Mounissamy, 2015).

Sleep paralysis

Sleep paralysis is a very commonly experienced condition (Sharpless & Barber, 2011), one that probably affects around forty–fifty per cent of people at some stage in their lives (Buzzi & Cirignotta, 2000). Most people quickly forget episodes of sleep paralysis and it is usually not considered a problem that indicates treatment. In others it can occur quite often and be a cause of some distress, as it is quite an unusual and disconcerting experience. Essentially all that is happening with this condition is that there is a slight mismatch in awaking from REM sleep. As we saw in Chapter One, REM sleep is associated with muscle atonia, or paralysis, and this is a normal feature of REM sleep. The problem in people whom experience sleep paralysis is that their brains have achieved wakefulness, but this REM atonia (controlled by the brainstem) has failed to "switch off", so the individual awakens, but cannot move. This very transient state only lasts for a few seconds, but, to the person experiencing it, these seconds can feel like an age and are often linked to feelings of distress (especially if they have been experiencing an upsetting dream just beforehand). People with sleep paralysis often describe trying to scream or shout, but without managing to make any noise, or to make huge efforts to try and move, but without success. However, no one ever fully wakes-up being permanently paralysed. This state only lasts for a few seconds and then the brainstem seems to kick back in and we lose our REM sleep-associated atonia. All is normal and well again, but for the anxiety experienced by people who do this regularly, which, most unfortunately, seems to make the problem worse. Over-attending to this condition makes the phenomenon more likely to occur, but the treatment is very straightforward and involves the normalisation of the condition, so allowing the client's anxiety about it to diminish, this is usually associated with a reduction in the frequency and severity of events and less distress in the person experiencing them.

REM sleep behaviour disorder

The most common REM sleep parasomnia is REM sleep Behaviour Disorder or RBD and is characterised by a loss of the normal REM sleep-associated muscle atonia. People with RBD can therefore move around, and sometimes move quite violently, during periods of REM sleep. Age of onset is in the range of twenty to eighty years and RBD may be prodromal for Parkinson's disease and Dementia with Lewy Bodies (Boeve, Silber, & Ferman, 2004). Again, we will look further into RBD in Chapter Six.

Periodic leg movements

Jerky limb movements in, and when going to, sleep again affect almost everyone at some stage of their lives, but in some people these movements can be very frequent, discomforting and prove to be a significant problem especially for the initiation of sleep. In the extreme, an individual may be diagnosed with periodic limb movement disorder (PLMD) with limb movements occurring in all stages of non-REM sleep, manifesting as twitching or jerking of the limbs, hands and/or feet, and causing excessive daytime sleepiness. As people with PLMD only move their limbs whilst asleep they may often be unaware that they are moving at all, and their daytime sleepiness is a mystery to them. As such, reports are often made by spouses or partners. There is no known cure for PLMD and so it is usually managed pharmacologically with benzodiazepine or dopaminergic medications (Aurora et al., 2012). Periodic limb movements (PLMs) can co-occur with restless legs syndrome (RLS), with many people who report RLS also having PLMs. Although the conditions can appear in isolation, with many people who experience PLMs not having concomitant, RLS.

Restless legs syndrome

Although related to periodic limb movement disorder, those with RLS (also known as Ekbom disease) may have the condition in isolation. The distinction between the two conditions is that RLS can occur during wakefulness, whereas PLMs occur exclusively during sleep. RLS can occur as a primary, idiopathic condition with a strong genetic element, or as a secondary condition to a range of disorders including: iron deficiency, diabetes, Parkinson's disease, fibromyalgia, thyroid disease, and attention deficit hyperactivity disorder (ADHD). RLS is a relatively common condition affecting five–fifteen per cent of adults, although there is a wide range of severity (Leschziner & Gringras, 2012). As with PLMs there is no known cure, although some relief can be found in leg stretching and other behavioural strategies, to which we will return in Chapters Four and Five. Management of the condition is usually made by the prescription of dopaminergic or benzodiazepine medications and sometimes clonazepam as with PLMD (Aurora et al., 2012).

The more unusual parasomnias

Sexsomnia

Sleep sex, or sexsomnia, is a relatively recent addition to the collection of parasomnias and has a range of presentations from mild to intense sexual activity during sleep, even being used successfully as a defence in several rape cases. As with the other parasomnias the activity is often unknown to the person who is experiencing the condition and reports are often made by partners or spouses. Feelings of guilt and shame are common experiences of people who exhibit sexual activity during their sleep when they are informed of their nocturnal activities. The exact number of people who engage in sexual activity during their sleep is unknown due to a lack of reporting as a result of this embarrassment and shame.

The successful use of sexsomnia as a defence in several rape cases, and indeed of sleep homicide as a defence for murder (see next section), revolves around the concept of culpability. People who have been able to demonstrate that they experience aberrant sleep patterns as defined by polysomnography (PSG), an abundance of parasomnias, a personal and family history of poor sleep and parasomnias, and guilt and remorse for their activities, have been acquitted on the basis of not being culpable for their actions as they were asleep at the time the offending act was committed. It should be noted that several people have also attempted to use sexsomnia and sleepwalking as defence for criminal acts and have been found guilty as they have failed to demonstrate abnormal PSG outcomes, a personal and family history of parasomnia, and guilt and remorse for their actions (Morrison, Rumbold, & Riha, 2014).

Sleep homicide

Perhaps the most famous (or infamous) case of sleep homicide is that of Kenneth Parks. Mr Parks drove approximately fifteen kilometres in his car, brutally assaulted his in-laws, killing his father-in-law and leaving his mother-in-law with severe injuries, drove home and woke up in his driveway. Covered in blood, but with complete amnesia for the preceding events he drove himself to the local police station. He stated that he did not know what he had done, but that he thought that he must have done something terrible, as the blood he was covered in was not his own. Police later discovered the tragic events of that night and Kenneth Parks was arrested and put on trial for murder. He was eventually acquitted as the judge considered that he was not culpable for his actions, as they were considered to be an automatisation and a complex somnambulism (sleepwalking behaviour), which occurred whilst he was asleep (Schenk, 2005).

There were a number of factors that came into play in the exoneration of Parks for the death and severe injuries he inflicted on his family:

- He had a good relationship with them.
- He was remorseful for what he had done.
- He had a history of aberrant sleep behaviours (sleepwalking/sleep talking etc.).
- He had a large number of genetically related family members whom also had aberrant sleep behaviours.

- He had an aberrant sleeping EEG profile.
- He reported no memory of the events.
- He turned himself into the local police station.
- He did not stand to gain financially, or in any other way, from their death.

These factors convinced the Judge that he was not culpable for murder as his behaviours on that night were considered to be a complex automatism and so were beyond his conscious control (Schenck, 2005). Since Parks there have been numerous homicide cases in which the accused have attempted to use complex somnambulism as a defence for murder. These "copy-cats" have often failed to meet the above criteria and have subsequently been prosecuted for murder. Usually, as these accused individuals did not have such a good relationship with the victim, they had something significant to gain from the death of the victim, and/or did not show a history of aberrant sleep, or a currently aberrant sleeping EEG profile, there may also have been evidence of premeditation to the crime, or memory of their activities afterwards.

Sleep-related eating disorder

Sleep eating is another example of one of the more unusual parasomnias and manifest from low level snacking in bed, to the full preparation, consumption, and even clearing up of a meal, sometimes involving the preparation of ingredients and even heated cooking. As with the other parasomnias people who eat in their sleep may be unaware of their behaviour and may awaken to find wrappers/packets in their beds with them, indicating their nocturnal eating practises. The condition is relatively rare and can lead to weight-gain and, because it is also a complex somnambulism/automatism, often being out-with the conscious awareness of the individual experiencing this condition, may be an "occult" precipitant to obesity. There is little evidence as to the effective psychobehavioural treatment of the condition, with dopamine agonists and the anti-seizure medication usually being prescribed. Topiramate has demonstrated the most utility in treatment (Schenck & Mahowald, 1994).

Exploding head syndrome

A rather strange and unpleasant parasomnia is that of exploding head syndrome, whereby the individual whom experiences the phenomenon perceives to hear popping or banging noises in their ears, particularly on going to sleep. Not much is known or reported about the syndrome, but it is likely an example of a hypnogogic hallucination (i.e., an auditory hallucination experienced on going to sleep), which can sometimes co-occur with flashes of light (Pearce, 1989). Essentially the condition is considered benign and, as such, extensive investigations and treatment interventions are not indicated, although some patients have demonstrated a reduction in symptoms of the condition with the use of tricyclic antidepressant medication (Frese, Summ, & Evers, 2014).

Sleep apnoea

The cessation of breathing in sleep is referred to as sleep apnoea, from the Greek for "no-gas". There is also a variation of this where there is reduced ventilation, referred to as "hypopnoea", or "reduced-gas", where the individual still breathes, but not enough to maintain blood oxygen (O_2) saturation levels (or to rid the blood of carbon dioxide (CO_2)). This increase of CO_2 in the blood causes the blood to become slightly acidic, a condition referred to as hypercapnia. During sleep, hypercapnia is recognised by the brainstem, which triggers an awakening to enable the individual to start breathing again and so excrete the troublesome CO_2 and replenish the blood with the required O_2.

The experience of the sleeper with apnoea is that (in extreme cases) individuals may stop breathing for up to, or even over, a minute and this can occur perhaps thirty to forty times per hour during through the night. The hypercapnia-induced awakenings result in a large gasp for air. This gasping is a key diagnostic feature of apnoea and is often noticed by spouses or partners of people with the condition. The characteristic gasping of people with apnoea rebalances the gas levels of the blood, but the individual may be completely unaware that they are waking for these brief periods to gasp for air. Such "micro-arousals" are often beyond the awareness of the individual experiencing them if the arousal lasts less than a minute. There are two very important considerations for the person with apnoea here:

- The continual awakening to rebalance the gas levels in the blood persistently knock the sleeper out of their all-important deep, slow wave sleep stages, leaving them with mostly light sleep through the night, so depriving them of much of their restorative deep sleep.

- As these awakenings are often very transient (microarousals are usually less than one minute in duration), they may often (or even always) occur without the awareness of the person with apnoea. So, even though they may have awoken up to thirty times per hour during the night, they may feel like they have slept continually.

The result, is that in the morning the person with apnoea awakens feeling terrible (as they have had very little restorative, deep sleep and have had multiple awakenings and very disturbed sleep through the night). They are also often confused as they feel like they have had a fairly undisturbed sleep. Further to this, they also experience Excessive Daytime Sleepiness (EDS) to the point where they may be unable to function effectively during the daytime even to the point where they can no longer work. The prolonged experience of apnoea precipitates significant loading to the pulmonary side of the heart (the part of the heart that cycles blood to and back from the lungs), eventually leading to chronic pulmonary heart disease. These can collaborate to significantly reduce the lifespan, and quality of life, of the person with apnoea. As the experience often occurs beyond the conscious awareness of the individual themselves. Apnoea is often reported by partners or spouses, and, as there are a large number of people who sleep alone, exact numbers of people with apnoea in the community is unknown, but are likely to be much larger than are known to healthcare professionals treating these conditions due to ignorance of the presence of the condition. Risk factors for apnoea include:

- Being male (although women are also affected).
- Being overweight.
- Snoring (the more extreme, the more likely to have apnoea).
- Having hypertension.
- Being over fifty years of age.
- Being excessively tired during the daytime, despite feeling as if enough sleep has been taken (Phillips, Cook, Schmitt, & Berry, 1989).

There are subdivisions of apnoea (obstructive and central), these will be discussed below.

Obstructive sleep apnoea

Obstructive sleep apnoea (OSA) is caused by a physical reduction in the aperture of the airway, this is often exacerbated when lying down to sleep. OSA affects four per cent of men and two per cent of women in the UK (Gibson, 2005). There can be various causes, for example, excessive weight around the neck, swollen tonsils, an enlarged epiglottis, etc. OSA is usually readily treatable. In the case of excess weight around the neck, then dieting and exercise to lose weight (both generally and in the neck region) can be very effective at reducing OSA symptoms. Antibiotic treatment of infected adenoid glands (or their removal) can also be very effective in the management of OSA, as can mandibular advancement devices (Lindemann & Bondemark, 2001) and rhinoplasty surgical procedures for epiglottal, or, nose, mouth, throat and jaw-related obstructions (McDonald, 2003). Often these approaches can prove very effective in the successful management of OSA.

Central sleep apnoea

Where it is possible to treat and "cure" OSA, central sleep apnoea has no cure, rather its symptoms are managed using continuous positive airway pressure (CPAP) machines. As its name suggests central sleep apnoea is a manifestation of a dysfunction in the central nervous system. More specifically the brainstem. Many autonomic functions are controlled in the brainstem (the cardiac, sleep and wakefulness, and the respiratory centres are all located there). In fact, the Raphe nuclei and the pedunculopontine nucleus of the brainstem, that are essential for the control and regulation of sleep and wakefulness are located very close to the respiratory centres. This goes some way to explain the pathogenesis of central sleep apnoea. Although the exact mechanisms are unknown, it is thought that the changing state of the brainstem as it phases through the different stages of sleep can, in some cases, interfere with these respiratory centres and cause periods of apnoea. As we saw above, this causes an increase in blood-borne CO_2 which in turn causes the slight acidification of the blood (hypercapnia). This hypercapnia is detected by the sleep centres of the brainstem, precipitating an "emergency" reaction that wakes the person from their apnoeatic episode, so enabling them to take on more oxygen—with the characteristic gasp of the person with apnoea.

As this phenomenon is occurring centrally (in the brainstem) central sleep apnoea can be considered to be a "hard-wired" condition and so remains, at the present time, incurable. The treatment for this condition involves symptom management with the use of a CPAP machine. These machines blow a continuous stream of air into the airway via the application of a facemask which is attached to the CPAP machine via a long tube. This air, as it is blown into the mouth and airway of the person with apnoea, keeps the airway open during the night and enables the person to avoid episodes of apnoea and hypercapnia. The result is that, sometimes within a very short space of time, the person with apnoea can regain their normal quotient of deep sleep (which may have eluded them for many years). As a result, their excessive daytime sleepiness (EDS) dissipates and they can begin to regain a functional life. Unfortunately, there is no "cure" for central sleep apnoea and the individual with the condition will be required to wear a facemask at night for the rest of their lives, in order to successfully manage the symptoms of this rather enigmatic condition (Bradley & Phillipson, 1992). Compliance with the use of CPAP is essential in this regard. Older machines tended to dry the mouths and throats of users and many found this side effect too much to bear, but more modern machines are equipped with humidifiers which help to prevent this problem and so improve compliance.

Catathrenia

Catathrenia is classified as a REM sleep parasomnia, although it can also occur during non-REM sleep and is characterised by a high pitched squeak or a groaning sound on exhaling (as opposed to snoring and apnoea which occur during inhalation). People who experience this parasomnia, like those with apnoea, are often unaware of the noise they make during their sleep, with bed partners often reporting the phenomenon. Some blood-oxygen desaturation can also occur during periods of catathrenia similar to those experienced by people with apnoea, along with concomitant reductions in slow wave sleep and excessive daytime sleepiness, which, again, can cause daytime dysfunction (Ventrugno, Lugaresi, Ferini-Strambi, & Montagna, 2008). Treatment for this relatively rare disorder usually involves the use of continuous positive airway pressure as with sleep apnoea (Guilleminault, Hagen, & Khaja, 2008).

Narcolepsy

Falling asleep uncontrollably is a fairly unusual condition affecting around one in 2,000 people in Caucasian populations (Dauvilliers,

Arnulf, & Mignot, 2007). The condition of narcolepsy is genetic in origin and affects not only humans, but also other mammals as well. There are two forms of narcolepsy: (1) with and, (2) without cataplexy. The loss of muscle tone associated with narcolepsy with cataplexy is the most extreme form of the condition and the one which most people will be familiar. In this condition people enter REM sleep very quickly and lose muscle tone, dropping characteristically to the floor as they enter sleep. Triggers include: emotional distress, humour, and even strong smells. Narcolepsy without cataplexy is the other recognised subcategory of narcolepsy and occurs with the same triggers, but without loss of muscle tone. People with narcolepsy have notoriously poor night-time sleep, with people with the condition often complaining of disturbed and unrefreshing sleep, and high levels of daytime sleepiness. As the condition is genetic in origin it cannot be cured, but rather the symptoms managed. The most effective and common treatment strategies involve sedative/hypnotic medication during the night-time hours and stimulant medication during the daytime in order to "enforce" a more usual pattern of night-time and daytime behaviours onto the individual with narcolepsy. Many people with narcolepsy are resistant to such methods as these involve consuming fairly potent and slightly toxic pharmacological agents continually throughout their lives and instead opt for more behavioural management strategies that have shown some efficacy (Ahmed & Thorpy, 2010). These behavioural interventions involve the scheduling of regular naps and rest periods in the daytime in order to stave off narcoleptic episodes and so preserve wakefulness during the daytime and consolidate nocturnal sleep. These require tailoring to the individual concerned, based on their level of tiredness and the frequency and intensity of their narcoleptic episodes. These interventions often take some time to formulate the most effective rest/nap regimen.

Sleep-state misperception

Traditionally not regarded as an insomnia or a parasomnia, but with new evidence suggesting that this condition may well have a physiological basis, sleep-state misperception, also archaically referred to as sleep hypochondriasis, often presents with clients entering the clinic stating that they have "hardly slept at all" or "not slept a wink last night", or "been awake all night". Even the most severe insomnia will result in sleep for a few hours each night, and so anyone professing to not sleeping at all is often regarded as exaggerating their symptoms, and are sometimes perceived by the treating healthcare professional with some suspicion that there may be some more underlying psychological processes at work. Often such clients can be effectively treated using the "shown discrepancy" method that we will discuss in more detail in Chapter Five. Recent work with clients who present with sleep-state misperception have been shown to exhibit uncharacteristic alpha and even beta and gamma wave activity during slow wave sleep (which is typically solely occupied by delta waves and some theta activity) (Finkbeiner, 2014; Garcia-Rill, Luster, Mahaffey, & Bisagno, 2015). This intrusion into deep sleep of the more characteristic "awake" alpha and beta waveforms may well explain the heightened arousal that these clients exhibit, often in the form of anxiety. Whether increased anxiety promotes the appearance of alpha and beta wave activity during slow wave sleep, or whether these waveforms in deep sleep are the cause of anxiety is yet to be determined. These recent findings indicate that sleep state misperception has at least some basis in physiology and may not be purely psychologically driven as was previously thought.

* * *

The previous sections of this Chapter have defined insomnia and parasomnia and identified the many and various forms of these conditions, such that perhaps the insomnias and parasomnias should not be regarded as singular conditions, rather umbrella-terms for the various forms of insomnia and parasomnia discussed above. Whichever form, or forms of sleeping problem a person might have, it is essential for the treating professional to identify as accurately as possible the type (or types) of sleeping problem that are present, but also to consider the "natural history" of that presentation.

The natural history of insomnia

As "insomnia" captures such a range of sleeping problems and conditions, and considering how any insomnia may develop, change, progress, or evolve over time it is important for the treating healthcare professional to consider this development and progression of the sleeping problem, or its natural history. Below in Figure 11 is a reproduction and expansion of Spielman's "Three 'P's" model of insomnia which summarises how insomnia can develop, progress, evolve, and become entrenched over time.

The first four of the columns in the below figure were first proposed by Spielman in the 1980s, the latter two columns to the right-hand side have been added to extend the idea of how insomnia progresses and is maintained, or entrenched within an individual over time. These Three P's as proposed by Spielman are: predisposing, precipitating, and perpetuating factors (Spielman, Saskin, & Thorpy, 1987). He argued that we all have some predisposition to becoming an insomniac, but many of us remain "sub-clinical" (as in the first "pre-morbid" column of Figure 11). Then some stressor is experienced, which precipitates poor sleep (the second "P" shown in the second column of Figure 11) and we overcome the clinical threshold and become insomniac. As a result of this precipitation of "acute insomnia" we may then begin to engage in behaviours which may not be conducive to good quality sleep, the so-called "perpetuating factor", the third of Spielman's P's. However,

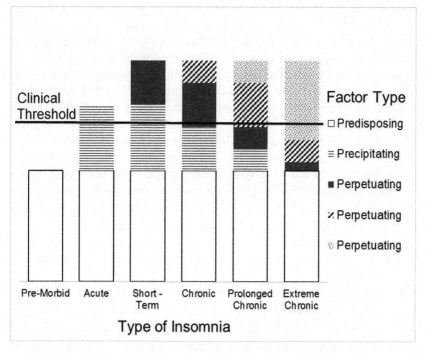

Figure 11. The natural history of insomnia from Spielman's Three 'P's model of insomnia.

over time we may engage in other behaviours, ones that are also not conducive to good quality sleep (additional perpetuators are indicated in the diagonally hatched and stippled bars in the fifth and sixth columns of Figure 11), and the original "precipitant" factor(s) may have diminished and perhaps even disappeared, or been forgotten, as in the sixth column, where the insomnia is being maintained by perpetuating factors alone. This idea is useful in terms of the treatment of insomnia, as it is important to identify from the patient the duration of the insomnia (i.e., to discover if the sleeping problem is acute, short-term, chronic or extremely prolonged), and also what the precipitating and perpetuating factors might be, or might have been, when they began, and how long they occurred for.

Here are a couple of case examples that illustrate how useful charting the natural history of a person's insomnia can be to inform their subsequent treatment.

Case example one

> Marjory is in her late seventies and has recently been bereaved (around twelve months ago). She used to have a very good experience of sleep, but has become more housebound after losing her husband as she cannot drive and does not live near to public transport. Her husband used to drive them to places before he died. As a result, she has become quite bored during the daytime and especially in the evenings, so she has taken to going to bed earlier to relieve the boredom of being alone in the evening. She drinks several cups of tea, and now occasionally naps in the afternoon, after her lunch, as she can no longer get out and about. She now presents as a little depressed and her sleep routine has gone awry as she is now taking a long time to get to sleep, she is often waking at around 3am needing to go to the bathroom and then struggling to get back to sleep.

- Predisposition factor: low—she had good sleep before losing her husband.
- Precipitation factor: bereavement.
- Perpetuating factors: (1) excessive fluid consumption in the evenings; (2) boredom, leading to napping in the daytime (reducing sleep pressure at bedtime); (3) boredom, leading to earlier bedtimes (leading to frustration about not sleeping due to reduced sleep pressure due to daytime napping); (4) increased depression as a result of

bereavement, and worry about not sleeping whereas she previously slept well.

Case example two

Terry is in his mid-thirties and has had a problem with sleep for the last eight years, since around the time that he was made redundant from his job. After losing his job his routine became much more erratic and he began staying up late into the night playing online computer games. After a while he began playing online poker and started to get into some debt. This affected his mood and he began to drink alcohol. Over time his drinking and debt increased and he became very depressed, which further disrupted his sleep.

- Predisposition factor: unknown, but probably quite low as younger people tend to sleep well (as a general, but not exclusive, rule).
- Precipitation factor: being made redundant eight years ago.
- Perpetuating factors: (1) An initial loss of routine; (2) a developing gambling addiction; (3) increasing levels of debt; (4) a developing alcohol addiction; (5) spiralling debt and alcohol dependency.

Writing these natural histories of clients sleep problems can help to provide a focus, and a sequence, for treatment and we will return to this in Chapters Five and Six of this book. Before that though, an examination of some of the cognitive models of insomnia and some current ideas about insomnia being a state of hyperarousal are warranted.

Cognitive models of insomnia

The natural history of insomnia, which was introduced in the previous section, has held sway for nearly forty years, and proved the test of time with respect to the pathogenesis and maintenance of insomnia, but it tells us little about the underlying psychological or physiological processes which may be instrumental in the development and maintenance of a problem with sleep. More recent work has begun to explore these processes and these will be introduced to form the conclusion of this chapter.

* * *

The first of the cognitive models of insomnia, which has received much positive attention, is that of the work of Dr. Allison Harvey, who has promoted the ideas of dysfunctional attitudes and beliefs about sleep, monitoring the self and the environment, engaging in unhelpful safety behaviours and selective attention, which are all key cognitive elements that interact to promote and maintain a problem with sleep. See Figure 12 below for a copy of Harvey's cognitive model on the promotion and maintenance of insomnia (Harvey, 2002).

Harvey's model has been widely received as one of the first truly cognitive models on the development and maintenance of insomnia. As such it suggests opportunities for assessment and intervention with people who are experiencing insomnia using a more cognitive behavioural approach: examining thoughts and feelings about sleep; reframing dysfunctional attitudes and beliefs; and challenging and changing unhelpful sleep-related threats and counterproductive safety behaviours. Below in Table 3 is a selection of types of monitoring,

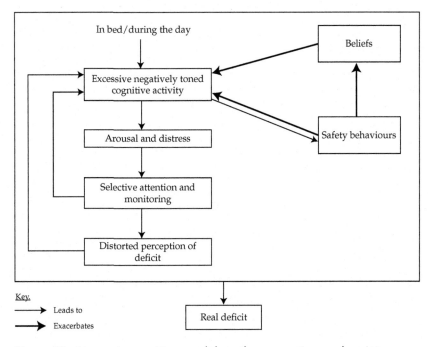

Figure 12. Harvey's cognitive model on the promotion and maintenance of insomnia. (Reproduced with permission).

Table 3. Examples of monitoring, sleep-related threats, erroneous beliefs, and sleep inhibiting safety behaviours (Reproduced with permission).

Examples of monitoring for sleep-related threats	
Type of monitoring	*Examples*
During the night	
Body sensations for signs consistent with falling asleep	Physical signs of "drifting off" such as slowing heart rate and loss of muscle tone
Body sensations for signs inconsistent with falling asleep	Heart pounding quickly, muscle tension
The environment for signs of not falling asleep	Noises outside and inside the house such as a dog barking or a neighbour arriving home
The clock to see how long it is taking to fall asleep	"It's 1.25am, I've been lying here for two hours and twenty-five minutes"
The clock to calculate how much sleep is being obtained	"Oh no, it's already 2am, that means I'll only get four hours of sleep tonight"
On waking	
Body sensations for signs of poor sleep	Heavy feeling the head, heavy and tired eyes
The clock to calculate how many hours of sleep were obtained	"It's 7am, I finally got to sleep at 2am and then woke up two more times, so that means I got about four and half hours of sleep"
During the day	
Body sensations for signs of fatigue	Heavy legs, sore shoulders, aching muscles, general feelings of fatigue, feeling "washed-out"
Performance and functioning	No energy or motivation, memory problems, concentration problems
Mood	"I feel so miserable, I've got to catch up on sleep tonight"

(Continued)

Table 3. (Continued)

Examples of safety behaviours

Feared outcome that motivated the use of safety behaviour	Safety behaviour	Consequence	Erroneous belief that is not disconfirmed
During the night			
"I'm not going to get to sleep because my mind is racing	Try to stop thinking	Paradoxical fuelling of excessive cognitive activity	Controlling my thoughts helps get rid of them and helps me to sleep
"I can't get to sleep because I'm feeling upset about the rude way my boss spoke to me at work today"	Drink a double whisky	Falls asleep easily, but poor sleep continuity	"Alcohol helps me sleep better"
During the day			
"I will not cope if I have too many demands on me today"	Have an easy day	Increase boredom and exacerbates daytime sleepiness, more time to worry about/be preoccupied with sleep	"When I haven't slept well I must take the day easy"
"If I go to the appointment with my client I'll perform badly"	Cancel appointments and take an afternoon nap	Unpleasant and/or boring day, more time to worry about/be preoccupied with sleep. Nap will interfere with the regularity of the sleep-wake cycle	Performance is 100% contingent on quality / amount of sleep

erroneous beliefs, and examples of some of the more commonly reported safety behaviours that are often engaged in by people with insomnia.

Another of the more recent cognitive models of insomnia has been put forward by Professor Colin Espie, one of the UKs leading sleep psychologists, who has conducted research in the area of behavioural sleep medicine for many years. His work supported the genesis of his Attention–Intention–Effort (A–I–E) pathway in the development and maintenance of insomnia presented below in Figure 13.

Espie's A–I–E pathway (Espie, Broomfield, MacMahon, Macphee, & Taylor, 2006) has gained, and continues to receive, positive endorsement as a useful cognitive model on how insomnia develops and is maintained, going into further detail of the subtle, more subconscious shifts in attention that are experienced by an individual with insomnia. This is perhaps most neatly demonstrated by one of Espie and colleagues' experimental studies which used a group of normal sleepers in comparison with a group of people with insomnia. Participants from both groups were presented with pictures which were filled with a range of items. Half of the items were random, innocuous objects

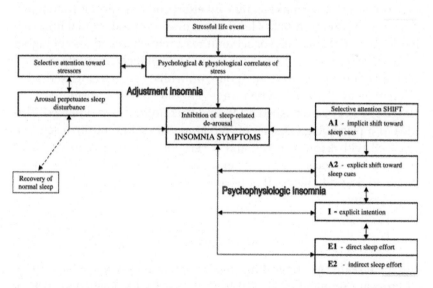

Figure 13. Espie's 2006 Attention–Intention–Effort pathway on the genesis of adjustment and psychophysiological insomnia. (Reproduced with permission).

(e.g., a toy car, a lemon etc.) and half were "sleep related" (e.g., a pillow, a bed etc.) All participants were unaware of the significance of the pictures in the study, just thinking that they were taking part in a memory recall exercise. They were then asked to try and memorise as many items as they could and then, later on, were asked to recall which items they could remember from the initial picture. Interestingly, the insomnia group remembered significantly more sleep-related items than the good sleepers (who remembered equal amounts of sleep-related and sleep-neutral objects), indicating a subtle, subconscious or "implicit" shift in attention to things relating to sleep in people with insomnia (Spiegelhalder, Espie, Nissen, & Riemann, 2008). Espie then takes this idea forward in his model by suggesting that, if people with insomnia attend to sleep subconsciously, and we know that they do so consciously (as this is one of the main things that insomniacs focus on), then they begin to start making some effort to sleep.

If one takes a group of good sleepers and asks them what they do to sleep, they will often struggle to describe what they do, as their sleep comes to them naturally, and without effort. People with insomnia, however, will be able to describe in great detail all the practices and rituals that they engage in on a nightly basis to try and attain this elusive, precious sleep. They make significant effort and this effort is fundamental in raising an insomniac's level of cognitive arousal, so making sleep harder to initiate (as sleep onset requires a reduction and loss of higher brainwave frequencies). So if one is in a state of high cognitive-arousal, with lots of beta wave activity going on whilst one is trying so hard to sleep, then the "relaxed" alpha waves associated with transitional sleep (stage one sleep) are pushed aside, and wakefulness is maintained. This idea of a psychological state of hyperarousal makes intuitive sense, it fits well with Espie's model and it certainly mirrors what we see in practice. The concept of hyperarousal also now has support from some physiological differences that have been found between good sleepers and insomniacs.

A state of hyperarousal

Recent research is suggesting that insomnia may well be a disorder of arousal (Reimann et al., 2010). Professor Celine Bastien's work on the electrophysiological differences between good and poor sleepers corroborates those psychological ideas put forward by Reimann, Espie, and others.

Bastien's most compelling finding in this area stems from some research she conducted using the electroencephalogram (EEG) and white noise generators with both good and poor sleepers. Any stimulus (whether awake or asleep) generates an "evoked response potential" in the brain. Such evoked response potentials (ERPs) can be captured using the EEG and manifest as a spike in brainwave activity. Bastien has been able to demonstrate that people with insomnia have greater ERP spikes when exposed to standardised levels of white noise whilst asleep than do good sleepers. These findings suggest that there is a physiological difference between the two groups, in that insomniacs are indeed hyper-aroused and respond more readily to external stimulation than do good sleepers (Bastien, Turcotte, St-Jean, Morin, & Carrier, 2013). This would help to explain why getting off to sleep and maintaining sleep may be more difficult for the person with insomnia and the old analogy of "hearing a pin drop" may well be a truism for those with a sleeping problem. Garcia-Rill and colleagues from Sao Paulo in Brazil have also identified intrusions of waking waveforms (beta and gamma wave activity) during sleep in poor sleepers (Garcia-Rill, Luster, Mahaffey, & Bisagno, 2015).

Collectively these findings suggest that insomnia can be usefully regarded as a disorder of arousal (Bastien, Turcotte, St-Jean, Morin, & Carrier, 2013; Garcia-Rill, Luster, Mahaffey, & Bisagno, 2015; Reimann et al., 2010). This idea opens up a number of potential avenues for further research and, most importantly, the development of efficacious psychobehavioural treatment approaches, which may begin to supersede our over-reliance on toxic pharmacological agents that have traditionally been used to manage sleeping problems in the developed world.

* * *

So far in this book we have examined the normal course of sleep throughout the lifespan and seen the various influences on our sleep, before a presentation of the insomnias and the parasomnias, we have also come up-to-date with some of the current theories abound in the pathogenesis and maintenance of insomnia and the potential psychological and physiological drivers of the condition of poor sleep. Collectively these theories have provided us as clinicians and researchers with the foundations on which to build a range of psychological and behavioural interventions for the insomnia population in the hope that previously relied upon, toxic sleeping medications will become a thing of the past. The next chapter of this book will therefore introduce the various assessment strategies that are available for the effective, patient-centred formulation of insomnia before presenting and discussing the various treatment approaches which have stemmed from the theoretical ideas presented above.

CHAPTER THREE

The assessment of sleep

The previous chapter examined the multifaceted nature of poor sleep and presented a selection of the more popular psychological models for the development, progression, and maintenance of insomnia. There are multiple methods for identifying the various insomnias and parasomnias, the most informative, as with most things, is to ask the person directly what they are experiencing and how they feel about their experience(s). There are of course other, perhaps more objective methods for examining a person's sleep and these will be the focus of this chapter.

Electrodes and sleep laboratories

The traditional, and gold-standard, method of assessing an individual's sleep is that of polysomnography (or PSG). This method involves the placing of electrodes onto the test subject's scalp in order to measure the electrical activity of their brain, the so-called electroencephalograph (or EEG), and other electrodes to record other physiological functions such as eye movements, cardiac activity, respiration rate and depth, and limb movements. These "many" electrodes, recording EEG and other physiological functions, provide the "poly" in polysomnography.

You may recall in Chapter One in the section examining the different waveforms of sleep that REM sleep "looks" like the waking EEG, in order to definitively confirm that a person is experiencing REM sleep and not wakefulness, we require the assistance of other electrodes to confirm: (1) atonia of the skeletal muscles; and (2) the characteristic rapid eye movements of REM sleep. Furthermore, in order to effectively diagnose conditions of apnoea, we require electrodes attached to the chest area to confirm the absence of breathing, and in periodic limb movement disorder and restless legs syndrome we require electrode feedback from the limbs. Figure 14 shows the typical electrode placement for the polysomnographic procedure.

So, in terms of definitive diagnostic criteria for the whole gamut of sleep disorders, the PSG method is the gold-standard, and the most widely applied, method. Most local hospitals have respiratory medicine departments that are equipped for the provision of overnight oximetry used in the diagnosis of sleep apnoea and so will have PSG capabilities. Every neurology department will also use EEG widely for the diagnosis of a whole range of conditions, including sleep-related narcolepsy

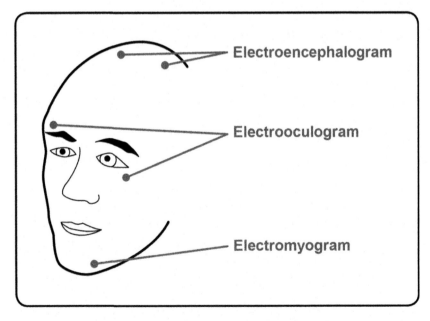

Figure 14. Electrode placement for polysomnography.

and wake-related epilepsy, along with the myriad other neurological conditions that are abound. The frequency bands for the different stages of sleep have been internationally recognised and applied to the study of human sleep since the late 1960s and, as such have pushed PSG assessment forward as the gold-standard method for the assessment of human sleep (Rechtschaffen & Kales, 1968).

Actigraphy

An alternative, less invasive and very useable and useful method for measuring sleep is that of actigraphy, also known as actimetry, or ambulatory monitoring. Actigraphy utilises algorithms to "score" an individual as either awake or asleep based on their gross body movements. Although very accurate in the detection of sleep and wakefulness, the actigraph cannot describe the various sleep stages, or delineate between periods of REM sleep and non-REM sleep (unlike PSG). However, the actigraph does have utility in both clinical and research settings for a number of reasons, some of which enhance its use over that of PSG. Below in Figure 15 is a picture of a commonly used modern actigraph.

First, there is a high level of agreement between the actigraph and PSG (above eighty-five per cent agreement in most populations that

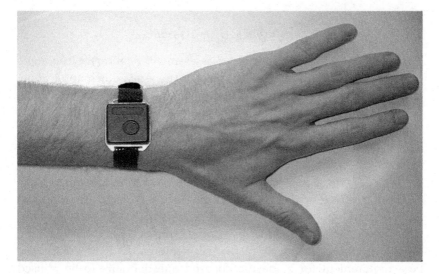

Figure 15. A modern actigraph.

have been studied) (Cole, Kripke, Gruen, Mullaney, & Gillin, 1992; Blood, Sack, Percy, & Pen, 1997); second, the recordings can be made naturalistically, in other words, at home rather than in the relatively strange setting of a sleep clinic where PSG is usually conducted; third, all data can be kept for analysis. Relating to this last point, in PSG clinics the first night's data is usually discarded as the client adapts to sleeping in the sleep laboratory, so-called "first night effects", which means that their adaptation sleep is not characteristic of their "normal" sleep and so these data are routinely discarded. Fourth, the actigraph can be worn for weeks, or even months at a time, whereas PSG is never usually conducted for more than two or three nights due to the expense of this assessment method; finally, and related to cost, the actigraph is a much more cost-effective method for the assessment of sleep, PSG requires specialist lab space, expensive equipment, specially trained personnel (polysomnographers) to operate the equipment and payment for these people overnight, which is costly (American Sleep Disorders Association, 1995). The actigraph collects data autonomously and can be interrogated by a trained practitioner (actigrapher) after the assessment has concluded and this interrogation can occur during normal working hours.

There are multiple benefits to the use of actigraphy, but the one major drawback is the lack of detailed physiological data on sleep stages, which inevitably limits its application especially in clinical settings.

Paper-based assessments

There are a multitude of paper-based assessments relating to sleep, some of which have specific uses, others are more general in their application, some have fallen out of common use, whereas others have shown durability in their application in the field of sleep assessment and research. Paper-based assessments can be broadly divided into three domains: (1) those designed to examine or probe a specific trait within a test subject; (2) those designed to examine the experience of night-time sleep; and (3) those which examine daytime sleepiness or dysfunction.

There is often some crossover in the domains which are examined (see the psychometric tests reported below) with some of the night-time sleep-related questionnaires also probing for daytime dysfunction (as this is a core diagnostic feature of insomnia) and there may also be a requirement for a specific, focused questionnaire to be utilised to answer certain research questions, for example, the Horne-Ostberg morningness-eveningness questionnaire that is still often used to determine the chronotype (lark, owl or ambivalent) of the individual under examination (Horne & Ostberg, 1976).

Reported below are two of the most commonly used psychometrics and an example of a simple sleep diary for the reference of the reader. These have been selected as a result of their extensive use and durability in the field of sleep research and their clinical application. There have of course been criticisms surrounding the reliability and validity of these measures, but it is not the remit of this book to enter into a lengthy critique of them, rather to indicate those measures which have known utility and those which have been most widely published in the scientific literature.

Perhaps the most widely used psychometric test for sleep quality in relation to the habitual night-time sleep experience has been captured using the Pittsburgh Sleep Quality Index, published by Daniel Buysee and colleagues in 1989. The test is scored into seven separate domains (subjective sleep quality, sleep latency, sleep duration, sleep efficiency, sleep disturbances, sleeping medication, and daytime dysfunction) and also provides a total, global score, any score over five indicates clinically significant sleep disturbance worthy of a diagnosis of insomnia (Buysee, Reynolds, Monk, Berman, & Kupfer, 1989). There has been some criticism about the sensitivity of the test, in that the global score should not be considered, in favour of scoring the seven separate domains that have been shown to load onto three separate factors of: sleep efficiency, sleep quality, and daytime dysfunction (Tomfohr, Schweizer, Dimsdale, & Loredo, 2013). Despite this criticism however, the PSQI has been used extensively in sleep research and has proven utility in clinical applications as well. Scores of five or more on the Pittsburgh Sleep Quality Index indicate poor sleep quality at a clinically significant level.

* * *

Another widely used paper-based metric in the assessment of sleep is that of the Epworth Sleepiness Scale used for the assessment of daytime sleepiness (Johns, 1991). Scores greater than ten on the Epworth Sleepiness Scale (ESS) are indicative of clinically significant levels of excessive daytime sleepiness (EDS). As daytime dysfunction is a core diagnostic feature of all the insomnias, the ESS has utility in the diagnosis of a problem with sleep.

* * *

Sometimes the collection of sleep information over time can be of particular use to the treating professional. This is especially true for exploring how the experience changes over time and provides an indication of the level of stability (or often instability) in a person's sleep profile. This can be conducted relatively easily using a sleep diary, an example of which from Professor Kevin Morgan at Loughborough University's Sleep Research Centre (UK) is provided for reference below in Figure 16.

* * *

An accurate formulation of a person's sleeping problem is essential for an effective treatment intervention (or set of interventions). As such, the clinician can get away from the "blunt instrument" that is sleeping medication and provide their clients with tailored treatment plans that are focused and sensitive to that person's needs. These then are much more likely to engender collaboration, promote compliance, and ultimately lead to successful, positive, and enduring outcomes for both the client and their treating healthcare professional. There is of course the added bonus of avoiding iatrogenic side effects so commonly associated with the chronic consumption of hypnotic medication.

* * *

This chapter has briefly examined a range of assessment techniques for the measurement of sleep, the "gold-standard" polysomnographic approach, another widely used empirical and objective method (actigraphy), and more subjective, self-report, paper-based methods. Each have their benefits and their drawbacks and usually a full assessment of sleep incorporates a combination of these approaches in order to more fully capture the sleep experience of the individual under assessment. The next chapter will examine the range of treatment approaches currently at the disposal of the healthcare professional for the successful management of their clients sleeping problems.

Daily sleep diary

Initials:		Date of Birth:			Date of Day 1:			
		Day 1	Day 2	Day 3	Day 4	Day 5	Day 6	Day 7
1	At what time did you go to bed last night?							
2	After settling down, how long did it take you to fall asleep?							
3	After falling asleep, for how long were you awake during the night in total?							
4	At what time did you finally wake up?							
5	At what time did you get up?							
6	Did you take a sleeping tablet last night?							

		Day 1	Day 2	Day 3	Day 4	Day 5	Day 6	Day 7
1	How well do you feel this morning? 0 1 2 3 4 not at all moderately very							
2	How enjoyable was your sleep last night? 0 1 2 3 4 not at all moderately very							
3	How active was your mind in bed last night? 0 1 2 3 4 not at all moderately very							
4	How physically tense were you in bed last night? 0 1 2 3 4 not at all moderately very							
5	How anxious were you in bed last night? 0 1 2 3 4 not at all moderately very							

Figure 16. An example of a sleep diary from Loughborough University. (Reproduced with permission)

CHAPTER FOUR

The treatment of sleep problems and insomnia

So far we have examined the science of sleep (Chapter One), types of sleeping problem (Chapter Two), and assessment techniques for the diagnosis of the various sleep disorders (Chapter Three). This chapter will now describe the range of treatment strategies available to the healthcare professional in the treatment and management of poor sleep. These can be broadly divided into the pharmacological and non-pharmacological approaches. So this chapter will begin by describing the various drug treatments available, before going on to explore the range of psychobehavioural and cognitive approaches for the treatment and management of the person with insomnia. One caveat though before commencing, and that is that the focus of this book is the psychological and behavioural treatment and management of insomnia. With that in mind the first section of this chapter on drug treatments will be brief, although it is anticipated that this will be enough to cover the main issues. Finally, a disclaimer, the author is not a pharmacologist and cannot speak with great authority on the mechanisms of various drugs. He is also very concerned about the over-prescription of sleeping medications. Although there are certainly circumstances and situations whereby the prescription of sleeping medications may well be warranted, there is most certainly an over-reliance on their use, both historically and contemporaneously. Part of the mission of this book is to promote non-drug methods for the treatment and management of insomnia and, as a result, the first section of this chapter will not be unbiased.

Drug treatments

The pharmacological treatment and management of insomnia has evolved over time, with older, more toxic agents being replaced by less toxic and more efficacious ones in recent years. The original sleeping drugs, the barbiturates, were very toxic and very dangerous in overdose. As a result, they were replaced by the benzodiazepine (BZD) drugs in the 1960s along with advances in pharmacology. These BZDs are opiate-based agents and, although highly effective, have been superseded by the more recent "designer" Z-drugs, which have less severe toxicity, tolerability, dependence, and side effect profiles than do the BZDs or the barbiturates.

Benzodiazepines

These agents have short-, intermediate- and long-acting preparations, the most commonly prescribed are temazepam (short), diazepam (intermediate) and nitrazepam (long). The shorter and intermediate acting BZDs were recommended for the treatment of insomnia, whereas the longer acting agents are usually prescribed for anxiety, panic disorder, and alcohol withdrawal. As these agents have sedative and hypnotic actions they are also used in the management of seizures, and for a range of other conditions requiring muscle relaxation. As with all medications there are the potential for side effects and the BZDs are no exception, with headaches and dizziness listed at the milder end, and with psychosis and convulsions at the more severe pole of the spectrum (although these are thankfully rare adverse events). There are however, other significant "problem factors" with these agents, namely toxicity, tolerance, dependence, rebound insomnia, withdrawal, and hangover effects; these will be discussed in the next few sections.

Toxicity

As mentioned above, the BZDs are opiate-based pharmacological agents (the same as codeine, morphine, and heroin) and as such have a toxicity profile that impacts negatively on the physiology of the person consuming them. Continued chronic use has marked effects on both the behaviour and physiology of the person consuming these agents. The most notable behavioural manifestations are increased drug seeking behaviour, and increased range of drug consumption. Physiologically the individual becomes dependent (see below) on the drug, there are altered neural pathways in the brain and changes in neurotransmitter concentrations (especially dopamine) (Mitchelini, Cassano, Frare, & Perugi, 1996).

Tolerance

After an individual has been taking therapeutic doses of BZD mediation for a while (a few weeks to a few months) they begin to tolerate the doses consumed and so their initial dosage becomes less effective. This often results in an increased dosage being consumed, and/or shifting from a milder to a more potent BZD. The chronic effect of which is that an individual who begins consuming a BZD will often, over time, begin to take more and more of the drug, and gradually shift from the milder (less toxic, less potent) BZDs with shorter half-lives, to more and more potent and toxic BZDs with longer and longer half-lives (please see the below section on half-lives for an examination of why these are important for the person consuming such medications) (Mitchelini, Cassano, Frare, & Perugi, 1996).

Dependency

After a person has been consuming BZDs for a while they become addicted to them, in exactly the same way as someone who uses/ abuses heroin becomes addicted. It is estimated that between twenty and 100 per cent of people using long-term, therapeutic doses of benzodiazepines will be dependent and experience withdrawal symptoms on cessation (Ashton, 1997). For this reason, these BZDs are not licenced for use beyond four weeks (it may well be appropriate for a short-term administration of a hypnotic to help a person to get some sleep during an acute episode of insomnia as they may be adjusting to new and disturbing life events (bereavement, redundancy, divorce for example), but use beyond this acute period is not licenced. Despite this the health-care professional will regularly encounter people who have been consuming these medications for *years* not the four weeks or less that is recommended, and indeed licensed for (Lader, 2011).

Rebound insomnia

Ironically, and most unfortunately, withdrawal from BZDs causes a rebound insomnia in almost everyone whom withdraws abruptly from their consumption of them. As a result, gradual withdrawal is required and this can take many months to achieve and the individual may well require significant levels of support during this time.

Withdrawal

There are also a whole host of negative symptoms associated with withdrawal from opiates, including (but not exclusively): insomnia, anxiety, agitation, dehydration, confusion, sweating, fatigue, loss of motivation, an altered perception of temperature, and feelings like one's flesh is crawling (Lader, Tylee, & Donoghue, 2009).

Hangover effects

One of the consequences of consuming a substance that has some effect on an individual's system is that this agent will be absorbed, assimilated, broken-down and, eventually, eliminated. The amount of time that it takes to eliminate a medication from the system is measured in half-lives, this provides an indication as to the amount of time that it takes for half of the consumed agent to be eliminated from the body. All medications have varying half-lives, with some of the BZDs having very long ones, and the Z drugs shorter ones (see below). The result then, of consuming a hypnotic medication, is that although it undoubtedly aids in the initiation and maintenance of sleep, but, with long-half lives, they are often still active in the person's system the following morning, leading to so-called "hangover effects", where the person's sleepiness is being maintained by the hypnotic medication at a time where they need to be awake (whilst driving to work for example).

The "Z" drugs

These have gradually replaced the BZDs since their initial release in the late 1980s through into the 1990s and early 2000s, although even still some people are being prescribed with BZD medications. The

Z drugs are a family of non-benzodiazepine drugs, which have less toxic side effect profiles and do not have such poor tolerance, dependency, rebound, withdrawal, and hangover effect profiles as do the BZDs. The mechanism of action of both families of drugs is similar, but the newer Z drugs have the benefit of shorter half-lives and do not affect the sleep stages as profoundly as do the BZDs, the latter of which tend to reduce the amount of restorative deep sleep, replacing this with lighter less refreshing sleep (Barbera & Shapiro, 2005). The most commonly pre-scribed of the Z drugs are Zolpidem, Zopiclone, and Zapelon.

Efficacy

There is no question that these families of drugs, the barbiturates, the BZDs and the newer Z drugs are all very effective at inducing and maintaining sleep in the people that consume them. They are highly effective in this regard. They are also very cheap to produce, and require a minimal amount of time to prescribe from the perspective of the healthcare professional. The industry is worth billions of dollars across the globe and the sale of hypnotic medication makes tidy profits for the pharmaceutical companies that produce them. Weighing these "benefits" against the issues discussed in the above sections with respect to toxicity, tolerability, dependence, hangover effects, and with-drawal calls into stark question the efficacy of the use of these drugs to treat and manage sleep problems in the insomniac population. The problem that remains is a lack of knowledge about, and access to, alternative treatment options which will comprise the remainder of this book. Unfortunately, very few healthcare professionals are trained in the psychological and behavioural management of sleeping prob-lems. Instead their training, textbooks, and computer systems, which are used once in practice, all direct the healthcare professional towards prescription of medication for sleeping problems. The National Insti-tute for Health and Care Excellence in the UK (NICE) guidelines do recommend cognitive behavioural therapy for insomnia (CBTi) as the first-line treatment for insomnia (National Institute for Health and Care Excellence, Clinical Knowledge Summaries, 2016), but unfortunately the healthcare professional then has no one to refer to for the deliv-ery of this treatment as so few people are trained in its delivery. As a result, they proceed to the second available option for treatment, which is hypnotic medication.

Half-lives

As has been mentioned above there are significant issues surrounding the use of hypnotic medication relating to toxicity, tolerance, dependence, withdrawal, and hangover effects, all of which are directly affected by the half-lives of these medications. The longer a drug is in the system the more of an opportunity it will have to be toxic to, and become tolerated by the system. The system will also have more of an opportunity to become dependent upon the drug and the drug will continue to have its specific (and side-) effects on the system until it is eliminated. Once eliminated, the system then recovers from the effects that the drug has had and there is a "rebound" towards the pre-drug condition of the system. For the hypnotics this rebound includes a recurrence of insomnia. As a general principle, drugs with shorter half-lives are preferable to those with longer ones in order to ameliorate this range of negative issues. With prescribers preferentially opting for lower dosages of milder agents in the first instance to achieve a desired effect; before progressing onto more insidious agents at higher doses, should the lower dosage, milder agents prove ineffective. Before we continue to examine the alternative treatment options for insomnia in the form of psychobehavioural interventions a final consideration of the half-lives of the more commonly prescribed sleeping medications is presented below in Table 4.

Table 4. Half-lives of the more commonly prescribed hypnotic medications.

Hypnotic medication	Usual dose (mg)	Half-life (in hours)
BZDs		
Diazepam	10	20–100
Nitrazepam	10	15–38
Temazepam	20	10–24
Estazolam	2	10–24
Z Drugs		
Zopiclone	20	5–6
Zolpidem	15	2
Zapelon	20	2

Source: *The Ashton Manual* (Ashton, 2002).

As can be seen in Table 4 above the half-lives of the BZDs are very long and the potential for next day hangover effects is high. These are less pronounced with the newer "Z" drugs, but there is still the potential for such hangover effects. As a result, the BZDs have fallen from favour and there is even parliamentary action in the UK to legislate for banning the use of BZDs beyond two to four weeks, currently BZDs are "not recommended" for more than two to four weeks of use (Lader, 2011). Many healthcare professionals will know well from their own contact with patients that there are so very many people taking these drugs for way beyond their licenced and recommended use, with significant negative consequences to them over the months and years that they spend consuming these agents.

Once you start, you cannot stop

As we have seen in the first few sections of this chapter on the treatment of insomnia, there are multiple issues attached to consuming hypnotic medications that have been identified. The problem for many is that once one has begun to consume medications for the treatment of insomnia then it becomes very difficult to stop. There are a number of reasons for this: first, there are a lack of trained professionals to deliver alternative, non-drug treatment options; second, and related to this first reason, there is a lack of awareness, in both the general population, as well as within the population of healthcare professionals, that other non-drug options even exist, and that for many, these are highly efficacious for the successful treatment of insomnia. Third, there is a progression with the consumption of medications, as we saw above, with increasing dosages and higher potency medications being utilised as an individual with insomnia begins to adapt to and to tolerate their medication. Finally, with the increased potential for side effects and hangover effects when consuming hypnotics, an individual is more prone to physical accident and negative psychological consequences, that may provide additional sources of distress and discomfort which have the potential to perpetuate their insomnia, thus requiring more intervention; a vicious circle.

* * *

With the multitude of problems abound in the use of pharma for the management of sleep problems, there is an increasing demand for less invasive, psychological, and behavioural interventions for the treatment of insomnia. A review of the evidence for the effectiveness of the latter, published in 2012 by Michael Perlis and colleagues, suggests that cognitive behavioural therapy for insomnia is at least as effective as medication, but that the effects of these psychobehavioural interventions may have more durable results than sleeping tablets (Mitchell, Gehrman, Perlis, & Umscheid, 2012). The psychobehavioural interventions for insomnia management are therefore presented in the following sections of this chapter.

Psychobehavioural treatments

The predominance of hypnotic prescription for the treatment and management of insomnia is unfortunate. For many years now we have well established, clinically efficacious, psychological and behavioural interventions for the treatment of insomnia that tragically remain under utilised. These remain mainly under used as a result of a lack of awareness in the community of treating professionals, as well as in the general population at large. Since the 1980s there have been a growing fascination, even obsession, in the developed world focused with a "healthy lifestyle". Such a lifestyle has almost exclusively centred on the type and amount of food and drink that is consumed, and the amount of exercise that is engaged in. The nutrition and exercise industries are worth billions. Sleep remains the poor relation in this triad. Regardless of how good one's diet is, or how optimal one's exercise regime, without good quality sleep one will not feel healthy, or be happy. Further to this, one's health and happiness will suffer considerably without good quality sleep, and yet very little attention is given to sleep. Medical students will spend a paltry amount of time studying the area and there is virtually no "industry" surrounding the delivery of healthy sleep; and what little there is out there in the commercial marketplace lacks credibility, is not supported by a well-researched evidence-base, and so is often regarded as quackery.

Again, this is unfortunate as we have the tools, and the evidence, in the form of very many well controlled studies, to validate the use of a range of psychobehavioural interventions that have begun to be branded as cognitive behavioural therapy for insomnia, or CBTi for short. CBTi comprises a raft of interventions that have been amalgamated into an intervention programme for the treatment of insomnia, and these elements have good levels of efficacy in a range of different populations: for people with psychophysiological insomnia; those with insomnia and depression; and those living with chronic pain. We also have emerging evidence for the effectiveness of certain of these elements in treatment of insomnia in children, older people, those living with trauma, and so on.

Indeed, the results of CBTi are so promising in these groups that there is no reason to assume that they would not prove at least mildly useful for anyone who does not sleep well, regardless of their particular situation or condition. Although extensive research is lacking (but emerging) for the extended range of clinical populations. The elements of CBTi include: psychoeducation, sleep hygiene, relaxation training, stimulus control therapy, paradoxical intention, bright light therapy, and sleep restriction therapy, and these will be considered in detail in the following sections.

Psychoeducation

The passing of information on the "science of sleep" as detailed in the second chapter of this book forms the base of the psychoeducation element of CBTi. Instructing the participant on the importance of: the circadian rhythm; the sleep homeostat; age-related changes in sleep; sleep stages; sleep requirements; and sleep types (short *vs.* long; lark/owl/ swift/dodo). This information delivery very typically forms the first one or two sessions of a CBTi programme.

Sleep hygiene

The next session of a programme of CBTi usually comprises delivery and description of the very basic sleep hygiene advice. This will be familiar to many, it is widely available on various internet sites, and has been garnered and shoehorned into multiple health programmes that touch on sleep as part of their programmes (e.g., the low-intensity Improving Access to Psychological Therapies (IAPT) training for Psychological Wellbeing Practitioners (PWPs) that is currently in-vogue in the United Kingdom at the time of writing). Indeed, most healthcare professionals whom have been out of training and in practice for a few years will have come across sleep hygiene advice and absorbed this by osmosis into the fringes of their practice. Usually though there is a desire for more detailed and in-depth information on the treatment of sleeping problems as sleep hygiene, in and of itself, lacks efficacy as an effective treatment for most people with a sleep problem (Irish, Kline, Gunn, Buysse, & Hall, 2014).

Sleep is affected by a number of environmental and lifestyle factors. Some of these are noise, temperature, light, exercise, diet, alcohol consumption, substance use/abuse, daytime napping, excessive time spent in bed, the use of the bedroom for activities other than sleep or sex, and irregular routines. These factors, which may benefit or impose on sleep, are collectively referred to as sleep hygiene practices (Hauri et al., 1982). Sleep hygiene consists of two essential elements: health practices and environmental influences (Bootzin, 1972).

Although highly intuitive in its detail, there is very little evidence to suggest that sleep hygiene advice is an effective treatment modality for insomnia (Irish, Kline, Gunn, Buysse, & Hall, 2014). Below in Figure 17 is a list of the most commonly reported sleep hygiene elements:

These elements, although intuitively sensible, lack any well-researched findings to support their efficacious clinical application (Irish, Kline, Gunn, Buysse, & Hall, 2014), with the exception of blue light (which predominates naturally in the mornings, with a shift in daylight towards the red end of the spectrum later in the day). The use of screens that emit light at the blue-end of the spectrum has been shown to impact negatively on sleep, and the rhythmicity of melatonin production and release, if used later in the afternoon and evening (Gringras, Middleton, Skene, & Revell, 2015).

- A comfortable bed
- A comfortable bedroom temperature
- Seasonally appropriate bedding
- Reduced noise and light in the sleeping environment
- Not exercising close to bedtime
- Not eating large amounts close to bedtime
- Avoiding caffeine in the afternoon
- Avoiding the use of "blue light" screens in the evening and especially in bed
- Not consuming medications, recreational drugs (including alcohol) that may interfere with sleep.

Figure 17. Elements of sleep hygiene advice.

Relaxation training

The instruction of the client in techniques that promote relaxation form another useful component of the CBTi process and there are a range of techniques that have been employed to promote relaxation in the client. Essentially these techniques involve what has been referred to as "a degree of withdrawal" and have included a number of practices some of which are listed here for reference: autogenic training; biofeedback; self-hypnosis; yoga; progressive muscle relaxation; meditation; mindfulness; deep breathing; and visualisation. There is little research evidence to support the utility of relaxation therapy, despite this it often forms a component of CBTi programmes.

Stimulus control theory and therapy

Stimulus control theory was first described by Richard Bootzin in 1972. With regard to sleep this theory states that sleep, although essentially a biological mechanism, is greatly influenced by learning. When positive discriminative sleep stimuli (i.e., environmental cues or conditions that are sleep promoting, such as brushing teeth and donning pyjamas) become unattended to, stimulus control is effectively lost with regard to sleep and insomnia ensues. This loss of stimulus control is proposed to contribute to both the onset and the maintenance of insomnia (Bootzin, 1972).

Behavioural, psychological, and environmental treatment modalities for insomnia are grounded in stimulus control theory and learning. Two such treatments have been developed to combat insomnia; these are Stimulus Control Therapy and Sleep Restriction Treatment (Morin, Kowatch, & O'Shanick, 1990; Spielman, Saskin, & Thorpy, 1987). Both of these cognitive behavioural strategies have been shown to be effective in the treatment of insomnia for younger adults (Chambers & Alexander, 1992) and for older adults (Friedman, Bliwise, Yesavage, & Salom, 1991; Morin et al., 1999). There is no evidence to suggest that some elements of these cognitive behavioural treatment methods may not benefit the sleep experienced by people with other conditions.

Stimulus control therapy (SCT) was developed from classical and operant conditioning theories and is one of the most effective psychological treatments for insomnia (Lacks & Morin, 1992). The therapy is based on strengthening learned connections between the sleep environment and sleep onset, and maximising the sleep promoting properties of the sleeping environment (Bootzin, 1972). The essential tenets of this therapy are to propagate the association between the bed, the bedroom, and sleep, to eliminate poor sleep practices, and to teach a patient with insomnia strategies for optimising their sleep experience by establishing a consistent sleep–wake schedule (Hauri, 1998).

Sleep restriction therapy

The restriction of sleep to induce a sleep debt in participants was first proposed by Spielman, Saskin, and Thorpy in 1987. The principle of this method remains well practiced and is often used as a strategy by the behavioural sleep practitioner in improving the sleep of their clients nearly forty years after its inception. The fundamental reason for its success and durability is its two-fold mode of action on the person with insomnia. First, the restriction of the time available for sleep inevitably reduces the amount of sleep of the individual under treatment, thus endowing them with a so-called "sleep debt". Or, in other words, turns up their sleep homeostat so that when they go to bed on subsequent nights they are more tired and therefore more likely to initiate sleep quickly. This is particularly useful for those people who have difficulty in initiating their sleep. The second, slightly subtler, but no less important mode of action of Sleep Restriction Therapy (SRT) is that it enables the client themselves to take control of their sleeping situation, empowering them to take effective change in the management of their symptoms by setting their routine of sleep restriction. This can be particularly potent in terms of maintaining compliance to, and therefore the success with, the programme. Further to this second element is the bespoke nature of the intervention, in that SRT is tailored to the specific situation of the client themselves, taking into account their usual (or preferred) schedule, whether they are short or long sleepers, and also whether they are owls, larks or the more ambivalent chronotype. These features further engage the client in the process as they are central to its design and delivery. The next chapter will detail the full process of SRT when we come to consider the treatment interventions that are employed in the REST programme.

Paradoxical intention

Adapted for use with people with insomnia, Frankl's paradoxical intention (Frankl, 1959) can be a useful technique for treating poor sleep and has been included as a psychobehavioural technique since its initial application for insomnia in the 1980s (Ladouceur & Gros-Louis, 1986). Several other well-respected groups have recommended its use for the treatment of insomnia (Morgenhaler et al., 2006; Morin et al., 2006). We will return to paradoxical intention therapy as a treatment modality for insomnia in Chapter Five.

Bright light therapy

Light has a significant effect on our sleep and mood, as was described in Chapter One of this book, with strong influence on our circadian rhythmicity and subtler effects on our mood. The application of bright light has been reported to have a significant positive impact on sleep outcomes in a number of client groups with links to melatonin production and vitamin D. With the exception of blue-end spectrum light in the evening from the use of screens that has shown to be detrimental to sleep (Gringras, Middleton, Skene, & Revell, 2015). Again we will return to this in detail in Chapter Five when we return to these psychological and behavioural treatments for insomnia.

Imagery rehearsal

The treatment of negative dream imagery has traditionally utilised the prescription of sleeping mediation, melatonin, and, on occasion, antidepressant medication. There is, however, emerging evidence for the efficacy of Imagery Rehearsal (IR) for those experiencing bad dreams, especially in children and those with post-traumatic stress disorder and depression (Nappi, Drummond, Thorp, & McQuaid, 2010; Thünker & Pietrowsky, 2012). The process of IR follows a cognitive restructuring method involving the re-scripting of the dream, and the rehearsing of a more positive dream narrative and associate positive feelings within the dream. The client is asked to discuss the content of their bad dream(s) and then, with the assistance of the therapist (or sometimes a parent), to write a new version of the dream which has more positive and less upsetting/frightening content, particularly focusing on feeling safe, secure, and positive within the dream and afterwards on waking. This new version of the dream is then re-read and rehearsed multiple times over a course of a few days, weeks or even months, in order to cement the new dream-course into the mind of the client. In time, the negative dream imagery is replaced by the more positive, and less threatening version and so the nightmares diminish in their frequency and severity. Often additional support is required alongside IR in the form of co-therapy with conventional psychotherapy for concomitant anxiety, depression, and or trauma.

Non-pharmacological management of restless legs syndrome (RLS) and periodic limb movement disorder (PLMD)

There has been an increased desire to manage the symptoms of RLS and PLMD using non-pharmacological methods due to the toxicity profiles of the common medications that have been traditionally employed for these conditions (BZDs, antidepressants, and clonazepam). Although research evidence is scant, there has been some promising evidence emerging for the use of a number of psychological and behavioural strategies for the treatment of these conditions. These strategies (including: exercise programmes, pneumatic compression, the application of near infra-red light, and massage) aim to improve the circulation, generate endorphins, and promote the production of dopamine. The number of studies examining these treatment modalities are few, but initial findings are providing some promising evidence for their application. There are recommendations to explore these psychobehavioural interventions in the first instance, before progressing to pharma, as a result of the poor side effect profiles of the traditional drug interventions (Mitchell, 2011).

Efficacy of the psychobehavioural treatment approaches

There are a large number of studies which have explored the psychological, behavioural, and environmental treatment modalities which have been successful in treating insomnia throughout all age groups and levels of cognitive functionality. According to a review of this research area conducted by Morin and colleagues in 1999, between seventy and eighty per cent of older adults with insomnia benefit from non-pharmacological treatments for insomnia and these interventions produce "reliable and durable changes in the sleep of patients with chronic and primary insomnia" (Morin et al., 1999).

This extensive review into the psychobehavioural management of insomnia has been corroborated again by the same group in 2006 (Morin et al., 2006); and the efficacy of these interventions supported for use with other populations than those with "primary" insomnia. For example, in those with sleep problems and cancer (Woodward, 2011); sleep problems in childhood (Tikotzky & Sadeh, 2010); older adults with insomnia (Montgomery & Denis, 2004); adults with depression and sleep problems (Manber et al., 2008); those with insomnia and living with chronic pain (Tang, 2009), anxiety (Belleville, Cousineau, Levrier, & St-Pierre-Delorme, 2011), and other mental health presentations (including alcohol dependency syndrome and post-traumatic stress disorder (Sánchez-Ortuño & Edinger, 2012)); and even some very positive results in an initial trial with clients experiencing persistent delusions and hallucinations (Freeman et al., 2015).

The limits of our knowledge and application

Although a large corpus of research evidence exists to endorse the effectiveness and utility of the range of psychobehavioural treatments for insomnia, there remain significant gaps in our knowledge to date. As a result of this there are a number of fruitful avenues for further enquiry in the field. Largely in the domains of extending our knowledge into the effectiveness of such treatments (and adapting these treatments) into more diverse groups of people. Especially those living with more complex physical and mental health conditions. There are various clinicians and researchers whom have already begun this work, but the evidence is scant at this stage and the research is still in its infancy. There is also some debate as to the effectiveness of the singular elements of CBTi (as this is usually delivered as a holistic treatment programme), with some criticism as to the lack of definition into the efficacy of each element of the CBTi approach (Irish, Kline, Gunn, Buysse, & Hall, 2014). For example, there is no conclusive evidence in the literature to suggest that sleep hygiene advice in isolation is an effective treatment for insomnia, so questioning the validity of its inclusion in the CBTi "package", yet every CBTi course includes at least one session on giving sleep hygiene advice. Again, teasing-out the effective elements from those with less potency is a work in progress as these methods evolve. The following section will examine the first generation CBTi elements and processes in more detail before we examine the initial, second generation CBTi package, the REST programme, detailed in the following chapter.

Cognitive behavioural therapy for insomnia (CBTi)

A number of studies from various research groups across the world have demonstrated the effectiveness of cognitive behavioural therapy for insomnia delivered by clinicians (Espie, Inglis, Tessuer, & Harvey, 2001; Morgenthaler et al., 2006; Morin et al., 1999) and trained nurses (Espie et al., 2007). There is also evidence for the effectiveness of computerised (Cheng & Dizon, 2012) and self administered modalities (van Straten & Cuijpers, 2009), although these latter treatment modalities have more modest treatment effects than those delivered by clinicians and trained nurses. There is also a strong argument emerging for the use of cognitive behavioural therapy for insomnia as being more effective than pharmacological treatment of the condition (Sivertsen et al., 2006; Mitchell, Gehrman, Perlis, & Umscheid, 2012), and that co-therapy, of CBTi and pharma in combination, as more effective than drug treatments in isolation (Jacobs, Pace-Schott, Stickgold, & Otto, 2004). We have already seen the efficacy of these approaches for use with a wide range of client groups earlier in this chapter.

Elements and process

The treatment process of cognitive behavioural therapy for insomnia follows standardised delivery of key elements including those described above of: psychoeducation, sleep hygiene advice, stimulus control therapy, and sleep restriction therapy and these will be presented in brief below in Figure 18.

An example of the process of a course of CBTi.

There are a number of different procedures of CBTi which have been proposed and below is an example from Professor Colin Espie in Figure 19.

Although other models exist (e.g. Perlis, Jungquist, Smith, & Posner, 2008) the basic process of CBTi follows that which is described in Figure 19 below sometimes including sleep restriction elements and

Stimulus control therapy

A set of instructions designed to re-associate the bed/bedroom with sleep and to re-establish a consistent sleep–wake schedule: (1) Go to bed only when sleepy; (2) get out of bed when unable to sleep; (3) use the bed/bedroom for sleep only (no reading, watching TV, etc.); (4) arise at the same time every morning; (5) no napping.

Sleep restriction therapy

A method designed to curtail time in bed to the actual amount of sleep time. For example, if a patient reports sleeping an average of six hours per night, out of eight hours spent in bed, the initial recommended sleep window (from lights out to final arising time) would be restricted to six hours. Periodic adjustments to this sleep window are made contingent upon sleep efficiency, until an optimal sleep duration is reached.

Relaxation training

Clinical procedures aimed at reducing somatic tension (e.g., progressive muscle relaxation, autogenic training) or intrusive thoughts at bedtime (e.g., imagery training, meditation) interfering with sleep.

Cognitive therapy

Psychological methods aimed at challenging and changing misconceptions about sleep and faulty beliefs about insomnia and its perceived daytime consequences. Other cognitive procedures may include paradoxical intention or methods aimed at reducing or preventing excessive monitoring of and worrying about insomnia and its correlates/consequences.

Sleep hygiene education

General guidelines about health practices (e.g., diet, exercise, substance use) and environmental factors (e.g., light, noise, temperature) that may promote or interfere with sleep. This may also include some basic information about normal sleep and changes in sleep patterns with ageing.

Cognitive behavioural therapy

A combination of any of the above behavioural (e.g., stimulus control, sleep restriction, relaxation) and cognitive procedures.

Figure 18. Psychological and behavioural treatments for insomnia. From: Morin et al., 2006.

Session one: Sleep information
Session two: Sleep hygiene and relaxation
Session three: Sleep scheduling
Session four: Cognitive approaches
Session five: Developing a strong and natural sleep pattern

Figure 19. An example process of CBTi.
From: Espie, 2006.

sometimes removing these for ease of delivery. In order to reach a wider audience and also to access people with sleep problems who might have difficulty accessing health care for, computerised and internet based CBTi protocols have also been developed, although there is variation in their design and effectiveness (Espie et al., 2012; Ritterband et al., 2009).

Efficacy of psychobehavioural insomnia treatment approaches

In certain areas there is compelling evidence for the effectiveness of the psychological and behavioural treatment of insomnia. A review of the area conducted by an American Academy of Sleep Medicine task force chaired by Professor Charles Morin of Laval University, Quebec identified eighty-five clinical trials which met their stringent inclusion criteria. These studies involved over 4,000 participants and reported that seventy per cent of these achieved sustained improvement in their symptoms of insomnia on both objectively measured sleep outcomes as well as on more subjective reports of daytime functioning. These collective studies reported moderate to large effects (not marginal ones), and a subset of twelve of these studies involved participants with other medical or psychiatric diagnoses, extending the idea that such approaches can have efficacy in the more vulnerable client groups (Morin et al., 2006). A recent and large review of the effectiveness of CBTi on a range of sleep outcomes has shown clinically meaningful effects on increasing sleep time and sleep efficiency, and at reducing wakefulness during the night and sleep latency (Trauer, Qian, Dpyle, Rajaratnam, & Cunnington, 2015). Computerised approaches have also shown good levels of efficacy at improving sleep (Espie et al., 2012), as well as improving concomitant symptoms of anxiety and depression (Ye et al.,

2015). There is interesting new evidence emerging for the enhancement of CBTi treatment approaches with additional cognitive and mindfulness-based therapy that has demonstrated increased clinical effects and maintenance of remittance from insomnia (Wong, Ree, & Lee, 2015). These findings open avenues for further research and development of the psychobehavioural modalities for the treatment of insomnia.

Limitations of the psychobehavioural treatment approaches

Despite the large body of research, extending back over several decades, supporting the efficacy of this range of psychobehavioural treatments for insomnia, there do remain limits to our knowledge and application of these methods. First, there is a lack of definition as to which of these treatments have greater (or lesser) potency, and in the ordering and organising of the delivery of these treatment approaches for people with sleeping problems. Second, there remains inclusion of elements that have questionable efficacy in the now favoured treatment approach of cognitive behavioural therapy for insomnia. The multimodal CBTi approach is in the process of being stripped back to its component elements with research on-going to delineate those elements which have potency compared to those which have less effect in order to design more effective and efficient treatments. This is a work in progress and will evolve over time to provide us with a better defined treatment approach. However, perhaps the most significant shortcoming of the whole discipline of behavioural sleep medicine is the lack of a comprehensive initial assessment procedures in the process of treating insomnia. Without a well-defined formulation of a person's sleeping problem (including its natural history and other "lifestyle" factors), any treatment will similarly lack definition, as a result treatment tends to follow a "standard formula", which will lack sensitivity and specificity for individual clients.

These criticisms apply to CBTi protocols delivered in research and clinical settings, as well as to those delivered via the internet. There is a requirement for the field to engage in better assessment procedures to provide specified, sensitive and person-centred treatment approaches, which will achieve a number of positive outcomes:

1. Treatments will be designed in collaboration with clients themselves, which, in turn will encourage compliance (and so more robust and durable outcomes).

2. Treatments can be selected from the available range, which are then appropriate for the individual and their experience(s), so saving clinician time and providing the client with what they need rather than inundating them with a potentially time-consuming and an excessive number of treatment approaches (some of which they may not want or need). This again will save clinician time, encourage client compliance and provide more effective treatment in a more efficient way.

Below are presented a few case examples to illustrate these points:

Marjory does not sleep well because she drinks large amounts of coffee in the late afternoon and evening.

Terry does not sleep well because he has a very erratic routine after being made redundant from work.

Mrs Johnson does not sleep well (but she used to for her whole life), because she is depressed after the loss of her husband and is frightened adapting to sleeping alone in a creaky old house a long way from her family and neighbours in a dark, rural environment.

A six-week course of CBTi would not be appropriate for these clients as Marjory needs some simple education about the effects of caffeine and its effects on the body and on sleep, which could be delivered to her in a matter of minutes. Terry needs some education about circadian rhythms and to talk through his thoughts and feelings about being made redundant. As a result, he would perhaps need one session to explain circadian rhythmicity and the importance of routine and then referral to a psychological wellbeing practitioner (or similar) for a few sessions to discuss his thoughts and feelings surrounding his redundancy. Mrs Johnson, who may always have slept well might need to have some sessions with a bereavement counsellor and some social support to help her feel safe in her isolated house.

Asking fairly simple questions of the client to identify what is happening with their lives surrounding their sleep problem seem obvious, but the current CBTi processes do not include these in their delivery. All of the above cases, and many others like them, would be shunted into a "standard model", which may lead a client to frustration and feelings of not being recognised, or their personal situations acknowledged. This leads to an ineffective and inefficient service and has inspired the development of second-generation CBTi models which can begin to address the issues highlighted at the end of this chapter. So providing people with sleeping problems a more effective range of treatment options, and also enable health service providers with a more efficient and cost-effective set of approaches.

* * *

The following chapter will detail the first of these new generation CBTi models, called the REST programme. It should be noted that there is no research to endorse this programme at the present time as this is newly developed and is part of an evolving domain, it is however based in the well-supported, evidenced, and respected arena of behavioural sleep medicine, but with the addition of more sensitive assessment procedures. The following Chapter then will describe the REST programme in detail; and it is anticipated that the interested healthcare professional, as well as the person with sleeping problems, will benefit from the information contained therein.

CHAPTER FIVE

The REST programme

As discussed in the previous chapter, although psychobehavioural treatment strategies for insomnia are known to be highly effective, and that CBTi is now recognised as the treatment of choice for a whole range of sleeping problems, there are some limitations to this approach. As a result, the REST programme has been developed as a second generation CBTi treatment approach, incorporating the elements of CBTi which have known efficacy, but with the added benefit of allowing practitioners to use the programme flexibly with their clients, tailoring treatment to the client in such a way as to:

1. Target their specific requirements more accurately.
2. Improve efficacy.
3. Potentially reduce treatment time by increasing specificity.
4. Adopt a more patient-centred approach.

These considerations can be achieved by making an in depth assessment of the client before developing their targeted and tailored treatment programme from the elements of the REST programme which are appropriate for them.

The REST acronym stands for **R**outine, **E**nvironment, **S**timulation control, and **T**hinking, and we shall examine each of these elements in turn in the following sections.

* * *

The four stage programme is designed to be used by some patients to improve their sleep by taking home information sheets and working on the recommended practices in their own time, others (those with more specific or complex requirements) may need the assistance of a treating professional to assist them with the information and recommended practices detailed in the four sections. This programme follows a "stepped-care" approach, recommended for use in the delivery of CBTi (Espie, 2009). This assistance can be incorporated into the other "treatment as usual" that a client might be receiving for other co-morbid conditions, with the REST programme being implemented in tandem with their current therapy. An additional benefit of the REST programme is that it can be delivered by any healthcare professional who has received training in their specific area and is suitably accredited and insured to deliver treatment to individuals presenting with the condition(s) they are trained to manage. Only a very basic level of understanding of psychology and biology are required to deliver this programme and such information can be gleaned from the first chapters of this book. An important caveat to acknowledge here is that there is always the complex case who will require more expert intervention. There is a responsibility of the treating professional to recognise the limits of their own knowledge, skills, experience, and practice; and so refer complex cases on to another professional who does have greater skills, experience, and knowledge for the treatment and management of these more complex presentations, should this be required. Some examples of these more complex cases are presented in Chapter Six of this book. It is anticipated that healthcare professionals whom have experience working with these specific groups may then begin to think about and apply the treatment approaches described here to their specific client-groups whom they have training and experience in assessing and treating. If there is any doubt in the mind of the treating healthcare professional it is always important to consider referral on, or at least seeking out supervision, and support, for the management of sleep problems in client groups whom they do not have extensive training or experience with.

Prior to the delivery of the REST programme a detailed assessment or formulation is made in order to identify the specific issues that the client is experiencing with their sleep. This is the first area in which REST differs from the original CBTi approaches, which traditionally do not place much emphasis on the specific presentation of the person with insomnia, only in so far as they do not sleep well. This detailed formulation is designed to identify which elements of the REST programme are then required, and so selected, for delivery (and in what order they might be delivered) to best help the client with their specific problem(s) with their sleep. This focus on increased specification again enhances and extends the REST programme beyond traditional CBTi approaches allowing the treating professional to be flexible, efficient, and client-centred in their approach. This enables the practitioner to deliver a more patient-centred course of treatment in a stepped-care mode of delivery (as proposed by Espie (2009)), which is therefore more likely to have better levels of compliance, and so faster and more durable results for the client than the more traditional approaches have done in the past.

The assessment tool

Below in Figure 20 is a sleep assessment form (for adult clients) that comprises the starting point for collecting information from the person who is not sleeping well. This then provides a platform for making a tailored and specified formulation for the efficient and effective treatment of the client's sleep problem(s). Based on the information presented in earlier chapters of this book the assessment collects information on: age, current sleeping routines, and preferences (i.e., long *vs.* short, lark *vs.* owl). The assessment then examines which type(s) of insomnia(s) may be affecting the client (e.g., getting to sleep, maintaining sleep, early waking, daytime functioning, and adjustment to environmental or psychosocial factors, etc.). Potentially maladaptive sleep behaviours are also then examined (e.g., caffeine, alcohol, nicotine and medication consumption, lack of exercise, fluid consumption etc.) Along with probes for, nightmares, sleep apnoea, and narcolepsy. Environmental issues are also explored along with an open section at the end of the form for clients to describe in their own words what specific issues they feel are impacting negatively on their sleep.

Please complete the following form as accurately as possible. If you require more space, then please continue on a separate sheet as required and attach this to the form when you return it. Thank you.

First Name:	
Family Name:	
Age:	
Duration of sleep problem (years/months)	
At what time do you usually go to bed?	
At what time do you usually wake up?	
At what time do you usually get up?	
Do you have a problem (please tick):	
Getting to sleep?	
Staying asleep?	

(*Continued*)

Figure 20. (Continued)

Waking too early?	
For how long do you sleep on an average night (hrs/mins)?	
Roughly how long does it take you to fall asleep on an average night (hrs/mins)?	
How many times do you awaken on an average night?	
For how long are you awake *in total* during an average night (hrs/mins)?	
Do you snore?	
If you do snore, would you describe your snoring as: *mild, moderate or severe?*	
Do you smoke?	
If you smoke, how many cigarettes (or equivalent tobacco) do you smoke per day?	
If you smoke, how long before bed do you smoke your last cigarette (or equivalent tobacco) (hrs/mins)?	
How many units of alcohol do you drink per week? (one unit = half a pint of beer/ lager or one medium glass of wine)	

(*Continued*)

Figure 20. (Continued)

Do you regularly drink alcohol in the evenings?	
How much liquid do you drink in the evenings (after 8pm)? (measured in pints)	
How many times do you have to get up during the night to use the bathroom? (Please enter a zero if you do not use the bathroom at night)	
Do you have any breathing problems?	
Do you have any heart problems?	
Do you ever sleep during the day?	
If you do sleep during the day for how long do you nap for on an average day (hrs/mins)?	
Do you ever fall asleep uncontrollably during the day?	
If yes, how often does this occur on an average day?	
Do you have any medical conditions that you think might be affecting your sleep (please state)?	
Do you ever feel too hot in bed (Yes/No)?	

(Continued)

Figure 20. (Continued)

Do you ever feel too cold in bed (Yes/No)?	
Do you ever have pain in bed which interferes with your sleep (Yes/No)?	
Do you have any bad dreams (Yes/No)?	
If you do have bad dreams, how many nights per week do you have them?	
Are you taking any regular (prescribed or unprescribed) medication(s)?	
If you are taking any medication(s), for what condition(s) are you being treated?	
If you are taking medication regularly, what is the medication called?	
Do you take regular (daily/weekly) exercise?	
What is your weight (in kg)?	
What is your height (in cm)?	

(Continued)

Figure 20. (Continued)

Is there anything about your living environment (for example bedroom or stree noise) that you think might be affecting your sleep (please state)?					
	1 = not at all 5 = completely				
	1	2	3	4	5
Would you describe your bedtime as regular (please tick)?					
Would you describe your wake time as regular (please tick)?					
Do you think that your sleep problem is treatable (please tick)?					
Do you feel tired in the mornings (please tick)?					
Do you feel tired in the afternoons (please tick)?					
Do you feel tired in the evenings (please tick)?					
Do you have trouble getting things done during the day (please tick)?					
Would you say that you are happy (please tick)?					

(*Continued*)

Figure 20. (Continued)

	1 = poor 5 = excellent				
	1	2	3	4	5
How would you rate the quality of your sleep (please tick)?					
How would you rate the treatment of your sleeping problem to date (please tick)?					
How would you rate your diet (please tick)?					
How would you rate your level of fitness (please tick)?					
How would you rate your mood (please tick)?					

Is there anything else affecting your sleep that you think might be important to tell us about?

....

....

....

Figure 20. An adult sleep assessment form.

After completing this assessment, the practitioner will have a good idea as to the specific issues of, and requirements for, their client. They will then be well positioned to tailor a treatment programme for their client selected from the elements of Routine, Environment, Stimulation control, and Thinking, as detailed in the treatment programme below. These sections are written in a format such that they speak directly to clients and can be given directly to them in a clinical setting.

Elements of the REST treatment programme

The first element is **R**outine

This element emphasises the importance of setting and maintaining a consistent routine. Clients are encouraged to identify a consistent and stable routine that is suitable and manageable for them; and then to begin to implement this in their day-to-day lives, preferably at the weekends as well as during the week.

The second element is **E**nvironment

This element emphasises the importance of optimising the sleeping environment in order to provide the best possible conditions for sleeping in; and reducing/removing any environmental factors that are not sleep promoting.

The third element is **S**timulation control

This element examines the behaviours and practices of clients and informs them about how certain activities/substances can impact positively and negatively on sleep. Particular emphasis is given to alcohol, nicotine, caffeine, exercise, food, and fluid intake.

The fourth element is **T**hinking

This element explores the thinking styles of clients and identifies the specific impact of low mood and worry on sleep, providing some strategies to manage these and so improve the sleep experience.

These areas will be expanded on in the following sections of this chapter. These sections are written for the lay-reader and can be used in the clinic by the treating healthcare professional to inform and guide their clients.

Routine

Generally speaking, good sleepers have good routines and poor sleepers have bad routines. Most adults sleep between six and nine hours per night, some are short sleepers (around six to seven hours per night) and some long sleepers (around eight to nine hours per night), but most adults will sleep for seven to eight hours per night. Some people also prefer to get up early and go to bed early (morning larks), others prefer to go to bed late and get up late (night owls), while some people are more in the middle (neither a lark nor an owl).

When setting your routine, it is important to decide whether you are a short or a long sleeper (i.e., what your ideal sleep time would be) and make sure this is realistic for your age. You also need to decide whether you are a morning lark, a night owl, or neither of these. This will help you set a routine that can work for you (it's pointless asking a night owl to go to bed at 9pm, or a morning lark to get up at 10am—they just don't like it and can't then do it!).

Only you know best about what sleep duration you like and what times of day and night you want to sleep, and when to get up; so you decide. When you do decide your routine, it is important that you allow yourself enough time in bed to sleep for the amount of time you want to, but not too much time in bed as this can lead to frustration and sometimes worry about being in bed and not asleep. You must allow yourself enough time in bed to get the sleep you need, but not to stay in bed for too long after your chosen sleep "window".

Once you have decided your timings you can start to implement them, it is important to get up at the same time every day (including weekends). If you cannot get off to sleep within fifteen–twenty minutes (or if you wake up during the night and cannot get off to sleep again for fifteen–twenty minutes) you must leave the bedroom and engage in non-stimulating activity, avoiding caffeine, alcohol, and nicotine and only go back to bed again when you feel sleepy. This may be around forty-five minutes later with the next circadian dip in alertness. A very good behavioural indicator of your circadian dip is the occurrence of yawning. Shortening your sleep time may lead to tiredness initially, but will lead to improved sleep on following nights.

Environment

A good sleeping environment will optimise your chances of getting a good night of sleep, but a bad one can seriously affect your sleep. Here are some general principles which may help:

Get a comfortable bed

Including a good mattress and seasonally appropriate bedding (i.e., not too hot in the summer, and not too cold in the winter).

Get some thick curtains

Sleep likes darkness and it does not get on well with lots of light, so some thick curtains, a blackout blind, or even an eye mask can help a lot in reducing light interfering on your sleep.

Look for ways to reduce noise in the bedroom or surrounding rooms/outside

This can sometimes be a bit harder, especially if it is a noisy neighbour that is causing the problem, but if you can find ways to reduce noise in the house or outside of it, use ear plugs, or even move your bedroom to a different part of the house away from the noise source (if you can) then these things can help to improve sleep.

Try to reduce "clutter" in your bedroom

People who do not sleep well tend to bring lots of things into their bedrooms, to occupy themselves while they are not sleeping, so they get used to going into their bedrooms to do things other than sleep (e.g., play on computers, watch TV, read, smoke, drink, send emails, play on iPhones/iPads etc.). Good sleepers engage in these sorts of activities elsewhere, and only tend to use their bedrooms for sleeping and for sex. Try to limit your activities to just sleeping and sex in the bedroom, and do these other things in a different room if you can.

Stimulation control

Often people will do things that do not help their sleep, some-times these things might seem obvious, but they can sometimes be overlooked. Below are some common behaviours that do not help with sleep together with the reasons why they are not good for sleeping. If you can identify any of these things in your own daily life that you could reduce or stop doing, then this may well help you to sleep better.

Drinking too much in the evening

Often people drink a lot of liquid in the evening times and this means they need to get up in the night to go to the bathroom. If you can limit the amount of fluid you drink in the evenings (particularly in the four hours before you go to bed) then this could help you to sleep through the night undisturbed.

Drinking caffeine and alcohol

Caffeine is a stimulant and will make it hard for you to go to sleep, so try to avoid drinking coffee, tea, and fizzy drinks (which have caffeine and sugar in them) in the four hours before you go to bed—or even longer if you can. People who really have trouble in getting off to sleep are recommended to not consume caffeinated drinks after lunchtime.

Alcohol (although it often helps people to get off to sleep, which is why many people like to drink in the evenings) stops you getting the deep sleep that you need and so you will often wake up early feeling dehydrated and unrested. Try to limit your alcohol intake to the recommended daily allowance (or less), try to have at least two alcohol free days per week (or more), and, if you do drink alcohol, try to drink in moderation, earlier in the evening, and not in the two hours before bed.

Smoking

Nicotine is a stimulant which raises your blood pressure and heart rate. As a result, it will make it hard to drop off to sleep and to get the deep sleep that you need to feel rested and refreshed. Try to avoid smoking at all if you can, for the proven health benefits that are well known, but, if you do smoke, try to avoid smoking in the two hours before bed, and certainly never smoke in bed as this can be highly dangerous.

Exercise

Although exercise earlier in the day is very good for health and for sleep, heavy exercise too close to bedtime is not good for sleep. This is because exercise raises your heart rate, blood pressure, and body temperature, these do not help people to get off to sleep. Exercise earlier in the day is really good for sleep as it makes people tired and ready for rest.

Eating close to bedtime

Eating late into the evening has the effect of raising our body temperatures as our stomachs get to work on digesting and absorbing our food. The sugars in our food are also absorbed quickly by our stomachs and the first sections of our intestines. These sugars have the effect of giving us a boost in energy, which also does not help us to get off to sleep. As a result, eating too close to bedtime has a similar effect to exercising too close to bedtime. In order to avoid this problem, try to finish eating at least two hours before bed and also try to avoid over-eating.

Importing sleep inhibiting items into the bedroom

People who sleep well tend not to have very much in their bedrooms, as that is where they go to sleep (as above in the section "Try to reduce 'clutter' in your bedroom" of this chapter). Conversely, people with insomnia, who "know" that they are going to go to their beds and not sleep, take things into their bedrooms to occupy and entertain themselves whilst they are not sleeping. Here is a major problem for these people, as, by doing this, they are only serving to make their insomnia worse. Preserving the bedroom environment for sleep, and sleep alone, is highly effective at promoting sleep, as entering the bedroom becomes a strong signal for sleep (in good sleepers without much in their bedrooms). Poor sleepers are primed for activity when they go into their bedrooms as they tend to be surrounded by lots of opportunities for avoiding sleep.

Making the bedroom empty of distractions helps to set you up for sleep, so try and remove anything from the bedroom that is not required for sleep, try to do everything that is not sleep outside of the bedroom, and, if you cannot get to sleep within fifteen–twenty minutes of going to bed, leave the bedroom and engage in non-stimulating activity until you feel tired (usually catching your next circadian dip, probably around forty-five minutes later) and only return to bed when sleepy (often when you start yawning). Similarly, if you awaken during the night and cannot reinitiate sleep within fifteen–twenty minutes, again, leave the bedroom and only return again when sleepy. This process forms a part of sleep restriction therapy which we will discuss later in this chapter, and is an important and powerful method for helping to associate the bed and the bedroom with sleep (which is what good sleepers tend to do) rather than with not sleeping and doing other things (which insomniacs tend to do).

Thinking

If you have low mood or are worried, then this can affect your sleep. For example, you may find that the same thoughts are going round and round in your mind, and so it can be very difficult to "switch off" and go to sleep. These are sometimes referred to as "intrusive thoughts" and are often negative in nature, and so can lead you to feel worried, stressed, angry, or upset. However, with the right help, it is possible to be able to recognise when you are having these thoughts and then practice some strategies such as "letting go" or altering the upsetting ideas to view them into a more helpful, positive light, so they impact less and less on your sleep (and mood in the daytime). People who are having lots of difficulty with intrusive thoughts sometimes require more specialised help and sometimes this requires referral on to psychotherapists, counsellors or clinical psychologists if that is what is needed. Below are some ideas that can be helpful.

If you tend to worry a lot in bed and this is making it difficult for you to get to sleep, or stay asleep, then try to arrange some time earlier in the day when you sit down and write on a piece of paper all the things that are worrying you. Then, when you go to bed, tell yourself that you have written down your worries earlier and that these can now wait until the following day. This will gradually help you to stop worrying at bedtime or whilst you are in bed.

The next day, at your prearranged "worry time" go through the list of things that were concerning you the day before and try to identify things on the list that you can deal with and then make a plan to deal with them (e.g., if it is finances, then arrange an appointment with a financial advisor/the bank). If it is something that is not that serious, then maybe you can cross that off the list.

If you have low mood and this is affecting your sleep, try to stick to a good routine, maintain a good sleeping environment and sleeping practices (from the other elements of the REST programme above) and set yourself some small, but achievable goals for the next day, for the next week and for the next month. These can be simple things like going for a walk, contacting an old friend, joining a group/team etc. These practices and activities can help you to break the cycle of low mood/mood swings and gradually improve your sleep as a result.

Treatment procedures

As stated earlier in this chapter, treatment can be tailored to individuals to meet their specific needs. The treating professional is then required to make clinical judgements, in collaboration with their clients (and sometimes other treating healthcare professionals), to prioritise treatment following the above four REST elements. Starting simply is usually the best course of action and, unless otherwise indicated (see below), the programme naturally follows a stepped-care approach, with simpler elements introduced at the start, and more complex elements then following sequentially (i.e., simple routine and environmental advice is then followed by the potentially more complex behavioural and cognitive elements in the "Stimulation control" and "Thinking" elements as detailed above. For many clients this natural stepped-care process makes sense and, if introduced gradually, can often prove successful in the rapid and effective treatment of a sleeping problem without necessarily needing to progress on to the more complex elements. For example, for some clients, just the adjustment of, and adherence to a good routine will be sufficient to "solve" the problems that they are having with their sleep. Thus the REST programme becomes efficient in that other, latter, elements are not necessary for that particular client. This improves clinical efficiency and negates the requirement for the client to engage in a protracted treatment programme, the latter elements of which might not be necessary for them. This stepped-care approach saves client and the therapist time, provides an efficient and patient-centred service and has been recommended as an ideal treatment protocol for the delivery of behavioural sleep medicine (Espie, 2009; Vincent & Walsh, 2013).

The sensitivity of the assessment process, as described earlier in this chapter, also allows for the treating healthcare professional to miss out elements of the programme that might be superfluous to requirements for the client that they are working with. Take for example someone who, at assessment, appears to have an excellent routine, but whom is waking often during the night to visit the bathroom: a very common presentation. Spending significant amounts of therapy time examining an already robust routine, exploring opportunities to improve an already good sleeping environment etc. will be inefficient, ineffective, and frustrating for both the client and their therapist. Skipping to the third element of stimulation control, however, and focusing on the amount of liquid consumed in the evenings, is most certainly what this particular client will need and the issue, potentially, will be resolved very quickly and without the requirement to spend significant amounts of clinical time exploring superfluous practices, routines, behaviours, and thought processes. We also saw three case examples (Marjory, Terry, and Mrs Johnson) at the end of the last chapter who provide other examples as to where certain elements of the REST programme can be applied and others missed out, as appropriate for these presentations. To recap and extend interventions for these three case examples:

Presentation one

Marjory does not sleep well because she drinks large amounts of coffee in the late afternoon and evening.

Interventions from REST:

Simple fluid restriction in the evenings may well be all that is required for Marjory, but seeing as most consultations range from thirty–sixty minutes it may well be worth quickly exploring her assessment form for other potential indications. Taking some time to reinforce the concept of a strong routine, and maintaining a good sleeping environment may also be worthwhile.

Presentation two

Terry does not sleep well because he has a very erratic routine after being made redundant from work.

Interventions from REST:

Obviously some time spent on determining a well-timed and appropriate routine is essential for Terry here and this may well take a session or two to explain the importance of regular timings, circadian rhythms, and establishing his sleep preferences in terms of chronotype and sleep requirement. During these sessions it should also be relatively easy to establish whether Terry's mood has been negatively affected by his redundancy and therefore to determine whether he needs to talk about this further, either within the current treatment, or through onward referral, as required.

Presentation three

Mrs Johnson does not sleep well (but she used to for her whole life) because she is depressed after the loss of her husband and is frightened adapting to sleeping alone in a creaky old house a long way from her neighbours in a dark, rural environment.

Interventions from REST:

Spending a brief amount of time examining routines and sleep practices is always worthwhile, and a good way to gently bring a client into the therapeutic environment with some fairly straightforward and non-invasive questions. However, it is highly likely that Mrs Johnson requires bereavement counselling, which may well require an onward referral. This could be conducted and treatment for sleep continued either concurrently with this, or at a later point in time after some bereavement counselling sessions have been undertaken, if this is then still required.

There are myriad other examples which could be made to indicate how the REST programme provides an efficient, patient-centred, effective assessment, and treatment approach. This is a step beyond traditional CBTi approaches, that often require participants to engage with lengthy multiple week treatment protocols. Furthermore, these potentially unnecessarily protracted treatment protocols will also interfere with (take time away from) concurrent treatment-as-usual for any comorbidity. Thus REST frees up therapist and client time to focus on their tailored sleep requirements, whilst providing space and time for the assessment, treatment and management of their other comorbidities.

Beyond REST

The assessment and treatment approaches described in this chapter thus far are based on those elements of CBTi that have known efficacy and will be highly effective for many clients. There are, however, some more involved treatment techniques that can be used for those clients whom present with sleeping problems that prove resistant to treatment using the REST programme. As such these clients might require more detailed consideration incorporating some other techniques already alluded to earlier in this book, namely Sleep Restriction Therapy (SRT), paradoxical intention, the shown discrepancy method, bright light therapy and vitamin D supplementation. These will be described in detail in the following section and comprise the next "level-up" in the stepped care approach.

Sleep restriction therapy (SRT)

First described by Spielman, Saskin and Thorpy in 1987 SRT has been used very effectively for the treatment and management of insomnia in a wide range of individuals presenting with sleep problems. As mentioned above in the stimulation control section of the REST programme, SRT comprises advice on leaving the bedroom and engaging in non-stimulating activity elsewhere, and only returning to the bedroom to reinitiate sleep when tired. This may often be around forty-five minutes later when the next circadian dip in alertness comes along. Again, if sleep remains elusive, the advice continues that the person again remove themselves from the bedroom and repeat this process until sleep does come within fifteen–twenty minutes. Important in this process is that a consistent wake time is adhered to *regardless* of the amount of sleep that has been achieved during the night. This sleep restriction initially builds up some sleep debt, that is, it turns the tiredness up on the sleep homeostat. Although somewhat counterintuitive, this sleep debt increases levels of tiredness the following night and, when following a consistent routine, should enable the individual with insomnia to initiate sleep more quickly and to remain asleep for longer. This serves two important purposes. First, it breaks the cycle of insomnia that a person may be experiencing, and second, it enables the insomniac to see that, given the right conditions, they can initiate and maintain their sleep quite well, maybe even as well as a good sleeper. These are the basic principles underlying SRT, but, as an adjunct to these there is an important outcome measurement and an additional element to the therapy that can also sometimes prove useful to incorporate, especially if progress with this initial, low-level SRT proves ineffective, and that is the calculation and monitoring of the person's sleep efficiency over time.

Sleep efficiency (SE) is a measurement of the proportion of time spent in bed asleep expressed as a percentage. SE is calculated by dividing total sleep time by the time spent in bed and this result is then multiplied by 100 to convert the index value into a percentage. The clinical threshold for insomnia is a SE of less than eighty-five per cent, that is only fifteen per cent of time in bed (or less) should be spent awake. If an individual goes to bed for eight hours and sleeps for eight hours, they will have a sleep efficiency of 100 per cent. If, however, someone is in bed for eight hours, but is only asleep for four hours, then they will have a sleep efficiency of fifty per cent.

The aim of SRT is to elevate SE to eighty-five per cent or above, and to maintain it there. Gradual reductions in the time spent in bed, to meet with the required total sleep time will eventually push this SE value to over eighty-five per cent. Should SE increase towards 100 per cent then this indicates that the individual is excessively tired. It is normal for someone to take between five minutes and fifteen minutes to get to sleep, and if their sleep latency is less than five minutes then this will push their SE above ninety-five per cent and indicate excessive tiredness.

So an ideal SE is somewhere between eighty-five (the clinical threshold for insomnia) and ninety-five per cent. If a participant's SE is above ninety-five per cent then this is indicative of a very short sleep latency, suggesting that they have an inadequate opportunity for sleep, thus the time in bed should be increased until their SE comes below ninety-five per cent. This process forms a behavioural experiment with the individual under test, to determine the right amount of sleep for them (Spielman, Saskin, & Thorpy, 1987). Adjustments to time in bed are usually made by thirty minutes on each occasion, and adjusted weekly, or every two weeks, although with more vulnerable clients this time frame can be extended to longer periods as required.

For example, Vallières and colleagues (2013) have defined a protocol for sleep restriction which is presented below in Figure 21.

The below example of a sleep restriction procedure in Figure 21 can be adjusted for different client groups based on their specific needs, or capacity to engage, and we will return to some examples of how the range of psychobehavioural treatments for insomnia can be adjusted for different client groups in Chapter Six. Before this though, some more examples of treatment procedures which have shown efficacy, but which have not necessarily been incorporated into traditional CBTi programmes.

Paradoxical intention

Although not usually a recognised element of CBTi, paradoxical intention is a useful psychological approach to the management of insomnia which has shown some good levels of efficacy. As such it is included here for the reader to reference its use as an adjunct to other approaches to insomnia management detailed in this book. Adapted from Frankl's logo-therapeutic approach (Frankl, 1959), paradoxical intention has been incorporated as a useful method of disrupting the behavioural activation system which surrounds insomnia. The person with insomnia will often make much effort to try to initiate sleep, and this effort raises cognitive activation and load, thus pushing sleep further away, as in Espie's Attention-Intention-Effort model from the end of Chapter Four (Espie, 2006). Paradoxical intention in the management of insomnia simply requests that the person retires to bed and then tries to maintain wakefulness. This, so often, is completely counter to the insomniac's usual behaviour that the thought process, being essentially reversed, disrupts the "insomnia activation system" and so sleep ensues. There has not been as much research into paradoxical intention as there has into the other psychobehavioural treatment modalities for insomnia, but there is enough available to suggest at least some level of efficacy for the method (Ladouceur & Gros-Louis, 1986). Indeed, there is reference, from well-respected sources, to this

Sleep restriction procedures
  (i) Sleep diaries used to estimate total sleep time (TST) and sleep efficiency (SE)
  (ii) Sleep window length = the average of the two last baseline weeks of TST
  (iii) The minimum sleep window duration is five hours
  (iv) Sleep window respected every night
  (v) Alarm clock used to ensure arising
  (vi) The sleep window:
       a. is increased for 15–20 minutes if SE $\geq$ 85%
       b. is kept stable if SE is between 80% and 85%
       c. is decreased to correspond to the estimates total sleep time if SE < 80%

Session 1: Sleep information and sleep restriction
  Aim: to transmit information about normal sleep, sleep disorders, and their effects and to begin sleep restriction therapy

  (i) Basic facts about sleep: sleep architecture, circadian rhythm and sleep homeostasis as regulators of sleep, and changes in sleep patterns over the lifespan
  (ii) Nature and causes of insomnia
  (iii) Introduction of sleep restriction therapy and determination of the first sleep window.

Session 2: Sleep restriction
  Aim: to restructure sleep so that it meets individual needs and develops a stable pattern

  (i) Review previous week
  (ii) Continue sleep restriction
  (iii) Teach participants to modify their own sleep window
  (iv) Clarify the distinction between sleepiness and fatigue

Session 3: (and following ones until sleep stabilization) Sleep restriction, developing natural sleep patterns
  Aim: same goal. In addition, teach participants to use sleep restriction

  (i) Continue sleep restriction
  (ii) Teach participants to modify their own sleep window
  (iii) Encourage fidelity to the new sleep schedule

Last session: Sleep restriction and therapeutic gain maintenance
  Aim: same goal. In addition, focus on further improvement and therapeutic gain maintenance

  (i) Continue sleep restriction
  (ii) Teach participants to modify their own sleep window

Figure 21. A standardised sleep restriction protocol.
From: Vallières, Ceklic, Bastien, & Espie, 2013.

treatment approach as a recognised psychobehavioural intervention for insomnia (Morgenhaler, et al., 2006; Morin et al., 2006). As such paradoxical intention enters the toolkit for the practitioner to consider for use with their clients who are having trouble with their sleep.

The shown discrepancy method

This approach can have utility in the treatment of insomnia and can be conducted in a number of ways, using either objective or subjective, self-reported measurements of sleep. It is well-known that the more severe a person's insomnia is, then the more likely they are to exaggerate their symptoms, particularly their time taken to get to sleep, their wakefulness during the night and to underestimate their total sleep time (Fernandez-Mendoza et al., 2011). The process by which this method achieves its objectives are through showing the client with insomnia that they are actually sleeping better than they think they are by presenting them with their own sleep data. This, in turn, reduces their levels of anxiety about not sleeping and they often begin to sleep better as a result (Tang & Harvey, 2004). One can use objective measures, such as PSG or actigraphy, or self-reported measures such as a client's sleep diary.

Bright light therapy

A now fairly long established behavioural treatment for insomnia is that of the use of bright light to promote the manufacture of melatonin to assist in the entrainment of the circadian rhythm (from the section in Chapter One titled "the influence of light"). The use of bright light boxes has been shown to improve mood as well being the recommended treatment of choice for Seasonal Affective Disorder (SAD). Bright light therapy has been used to promote sleep in vulnerable groups with small to medium effects (van Maanen, Meijer, van der Heijden, & Oort, 2015); as has the direct prescription of melatonin in normally developing, and in more vulnerable, children with sleeping problems (Bruni et al., 2015), and older people with dementia (Xu et al., 2015). There are a number of bright light therapy devices available on the market and these can be bought for around £100–£200. Protocols vary, but usually the client is required to sit fairly close to the device for thirty–ninety minutes with their eyes open. Light pressure (measured in lux see section "the influence of light" in Chapter One) again varies across devices with the more light pressure (and the more blue the light) having the most benefits. However, it should be remembered that there is very high powered light source available to us all, that is, the sun, which is freely available. All we need to do is to spend some time outside, preferably in the mornings when natural daylight is more towards the blue end of the spectrum.

Interesting developments in the world of vitamin D

One of the effects of exposure to natural daylight is the production of vitamin D_3 in our skin, that can then be used by our bodies in a variety of ways, especially in bone development and repair, as well as at a cellular level. Very recent work has identified this steroid hormone as a potentially key mediator in sleep that has potential for use in the treatment of insomnia. A large study of older men in the USA investigating the role of melatonin on sleep also measured a range of other hormones (including vitamin D_3) and noted that those with lower levels of vitamin D_3 also had disturbed sleep and shortened sleep times (Massa et al., 2015). There have also been some initial pilot studies which have shown improvements in sleep resulting from vitamin D_3 supplementation in adult populations (Gominak & Stumpf, 2012), and in those living with chronic pain (Huang, Shah, Long, Crankshaw, & Tanphysicianricha, 2013). These initial findings are interesting and exciting, potentially opening a whole new avenue for the treatment and management of sleep problems in a range of client groups, with the use of more naturally occurring agents as opposed to a reliance on toxic, synthetic mediations. Further to this are the range of simple and easily achievable behavioural techniques that have the potential to improve sleep, which may only amount to a focus on dietary intake (oily fish are a good source of dietary vitamin D_3) and exposure to natural daylight. Thus offering the healthcare professional strategies that are easy for the clients to engage with and that feel more natural for them, again aiding in avoiding the prescription of potentially toxic and addictive medications.

Summary

The assessment and treatment protocols identified in this chapter provide the current state-of-the-art in the psychological and behavioural management of insomnia, with well-evidenced efficacy for those presenting with poor sleep. First generation CBTi models, although known to be highly effective across a range of normal and clinical groups of all ages, have the potential to be more efficacious with the inclusion of sensitive assessment procedures preceding more tailored treatment approaches. Research is required to test this efficacy and to extend the use of these methods into a wider range of client groups. As such, second generation CBTi models such as the REST programme detailed in this chapter are beginning to be used in practice. The following chapter will examine the potential application of REST and associated psychological and behavioural treatments for a range of additional populations notably those presenting with more complex physical and/or mental health conditions.

CHAPTER SIX

Considerations for vulnerable groups

The previous chapter detailed the REST programme, which, based on well-evidenced CBTi approaches, can be highly effective at the treatment and management of insomnia in people who are otherwise in good health. There are, however, considerations which need to be made for people who have more complex needs, based on their age and/or any accompanying medical or psychological comorbidities.

As a general rule, the principles outlined in the REST programme in Chapter Five of this book are known to be effective for certain groups (especially adults with poor sleep, some older people, children, those living with depression, anxiety, or chronic pain), and there is emerging evidence for some other conditions as well, such as people living with dementia, trauma, and those who have had a head injury. In these more vulnerable groups, the REST programme may well need some adjustment to suit the requirements of the person depending on their situation and that is the focus of this chapter, beginning with adjustments and considerations for older and then younger people, before examining alterations that might be appropriate for people living with specific medical or psychological conditions. The list is not exhaustive, but has been written in such a way as to capture the majority of the more common presentations; and to signpost the way in which the approach can be tailored for others not specifically mentioned here. For those clients not specifically mentioned in this chapter, then adjustments which are made sensibly, inline with those described here, and with keeping the individual and their requirements in mind, are a useful starting point. However, if there is any uncertainty then one should always proceed gradually and with caution, and also seek the advice of a more experienced professional where necessary. This is certainly the case when working with children, those who lack capacity, or those who are particularly vulnerable due to an extremely pronounced psychological or medical condition, for example those living with brain injuries, dementia, or psychosis.

Older people

You will remember from Chapter One that as we age our sleep gets lighter as the bundles of neurons in our brains which control sleep and wakefulness, and the shifting between the different stages of sleep, do not function as effectively as they used to as when we were younger. As a result, older people have lighter sleep that is more easily disturbed. There is also an age-associate weakening of the sphincter muscles around the urethra which leads from the bladder causing an increased urge to rise and go to the bathroom during the night as we get older. Usually these arousals occur at a circadian peak, and it is often very common for older people to complain about difficulties in reinitiating sleep during the night; often because they have to wait for around forty-five minutes to catch their next circadian dip in order to get back to sleep. Worse still, if the arousal occurs later in the night (as again is often the case), then much sleep pressure will have been relieved during the first half of the night and so the re-initiation of sleep is again made difficult. This is the case as the sleep homeostat may have nearly reset to zero during the first hours of the nights' sleep so providing minimal sleep drive towards the end of the night.

Another common feature of getting older is that of retirement from work. This can be a very positive experience for many people, but for others it can lead to boredom, social isolation, and a reduction in self-esteem. It is not uncommon for people to begin to start napping during the daytime, so reducing their sleep pressure at bedtime, and also reducing their overall night-time sleep requirement which will be reduced by the amount of sleep taken during the daytime.

Bereavement is also a common experience of advanced age, bringing with it a host of social, psychological, and emotional sequelae that can have a negative impact on sleep.

All these factors can conspire to induce a sleep problem in an older person, so making the job of the treating sleep professional harder as a result of the need to probe for these types of activities, behaviours, and experiences of their clients and so be able to formulate an accurate assessment for them. Take for example the case of Marjory:

Marjory, who is seventy-four, in good health, but recently lost her husband of forty years to a heart attack around six months ago. They used to be active members of the community, regularly going out together to functions and events in their surrounding area. However, Marjory cannot drive as her husband always drove them to places. Consequently, Marjory has become relatively confined to her house, she misses her husband and isn't getting the stimulation (social and physical) that she used to get when she went out with her husband. She becomes bored and starts napping in the afternoons after lunch, and also starts to go to bed earlier as a result of boredom and finding quiet evenings without her husband around the most depressing time of the day. She used to regularly go to bed at 10.30pm and sleep well until 6.30am (a total of eight hours), but now she goes to bed at 9pm and wakes at 4am (a total of seven hours), but she also now naps for one hour after lunch (adding to a total of eight hours in every twenty-four-hour period). Her mood is low as she misses her husband and her former social life, but she is also perplexed that she is waking so early in the morning, something that she has never done before and something which worries her. So she visits her physician, who is very busy and does not have much time to fully explore Marjory's situation. He looks on his computer for preferred treatment options and sees CBTi as a first-line recommendation. Unfortunately, there is no one for her physician to refer her onto for this, as there isn't anyone trained to deliver CBTi in her region and so he looks up the next available treatment option and prescribes Marjory with 5 mg of Zopiclone. Dutifully Marjory takes her Zopiclone, and it helps her get to sleep a bit more quickly and she doesn't wake up until 5am, but she feels groggy the next morning and, in her daze, trips, falls down the stairs and breaks her hip. The replacement hip operation and the long recovery, associated with much reduced mobility, leads to more napping, more chronically disturbed sleep, lower mood, and an increased amount of hypnotic medication being prescribed and consumed. All of which would have been unnecessary if Marjory's physician had had a bit more time to spend asking the right questions of her, and/or having had someone trained in the delivery of CBTi to refer her on to. In fact, she was getting eight hours of sleep in every twenty-four-hour period both before and after losing her husband, indicating that there was no problem with her sleep!

There are many Marjorys (and Malcoms like her) up and down the country. They may have different back-stories, and their endings might not be so bleak, but there are many people being prescribed with hypnotics unnecessarily and, especially for older people, this may be due to normal age-related changes in sleep as well as behavioural changes during the day resulting from retirement, illness/incapacity, or bereavement. The interplay of physical, psychological, social, and environmental factors can be complex and it can take time and skill to explore these interactions sensitively and effectively. A couple of golden rules for advising clients here: (1) avoid napping, and (2) keep as physically and socially active as possible during the daytime, preferably out of doors.

Exploring the history and current experiences of older people as they present is essential in teasing out which issues are central to a sleep problem, and these can be usefully and effectively treated using the principles of the REST programme. It may be necessary to introduce interventions more gradually and also to think more broadly about enlisting the support and help of others in managing any interventions, for example family, friends, and other treating professionals. This is especially the case for older people whom are experiencing memory problems and those providing care for them, and we will return to these groups of people in more details in sections J and K of this chapter, respectively. Before then, a few considerations for those at the other end of the age spectrum.

Younger people

The sleep of children and the treatment and management of their sleep is a book in its own right and there are myriad publications sold every year in their millions relating to child sleep. Some are multi-million pound bestsellers, but few have much scientific credibility. One that has the most credibility, is extensively researched and employs evidence-based interventions is that of Dr. Richard Ferber, entitled: *Solve Your Child's Sleep Problem* (Ferber, 2013), and for the interested reader in this area this book comes highly recommended.

The psychobehavioural treatment of sleep problems has shown much efficacy in managing sleep onset and sleep maintenance insomnias and have been proposed for use with the management and treatment of the parasomnias (e.g., bruxism, somnambulism, nightmares, night terrors, and Somniloquy). Although there is a lack of detailed research for their use with these conditions emerging research evidence is proving promising (Sadeh, 2005).

That said, there are a few special considerations, that are worthy of mention here, when working with children who are having problems with their sleep. First and foremost is to consider the age of the child. As we saw in Chapter One, sleep requirements change as we age, and these changes are never more pronounced than in childhood. In attempting to determine the amount of sleep a child may require (and the number of naps they might need during the daytime), then establishing the age of the child is essential. Comparing this with the actual amount taken can be very informative. It is not uncommon to meet parents who believe that eight hours of sleep is enough for their six-year-old child. Which brings us to the second major consideration in working with a child who has a problem with their sleep, and that is: engagement with the child's parents or carers. Depending on the age of the child it can be very difficult to elicit reliable information regarding the amount and timing of sleep from the child themselves, and so, as with many other disciplines, it is necessary to glean such information from a parent or carer, and to develop and deliver a treatment strategy with their involvement and consent.

Two of the most common presentations with respect to child sleep is that of the occurrence of nightmares and sleepwalking. These often co-present and are very common between the ages of six to ten years of age, especially at times of heightened stress. In children, this stress usually results from: (1) trauma of some kind (e.g., an accident or abuse); (2) the separation of the child's parents and the subsequent upheaval of the home environment; (3) exam stress in older children; or (4) changing schools (moving from the relative safety and security of the small primary school where the child is the "big fish in the small pond" into the much larger, threatening and frightening environment of "big school" with many more children around, most of whom are much bigger than the child, and with (perhaps) less attentive teachers (as they have to deal with so many more children)). September to December of the first term of secondary school is a very common time for anxiety-associated nightmares to appear in children, and these often abate within a few months as the child adapts to their new environment.

Often identifying and working with the underlying trauma, stress, upset, anxiety etc. is effective in reducing the frequency and severity of nightmares and other parasomnias that are common in childhood (see Chapter Two), but there is one method that has been shown to be highly effective in treating nightmares in children (and beginning to show efficacy in people with depression and post-traumatic stress disorder who experience negative dream imagery) and that is of Imagery Rehearsal (Nappi, Drummond, Thorp, & McQuaid, 2010; Thünker & Pietrowsky, 2012), described in Chapter Four.

Another sleep issue relating to children, and particularly their parents, is that of encouraging a child to sleep by themselves and not to require the intervention of an adult to initiate and maintain their sleep. This is a challenge for all parents in the early months and years of the life of their child. The completely dependent baby does require multiple interventions through the night to feed, clean, and resettle. The infant gets used to this attention, but the parents naturally want their child to sleep through the night as soon as possible so that they can get good quality sleep and rest for themselves. Herein lies the challenge: breaking the child's association with night-time parental attention as they reach an age where they can sleep through the night by themselves (this is usually possible from about six months of age in a healthy child). Becoming independent in this regard is difficult for the child (who is too young to understand why the "usual" night-time attention is being withdrawn) and difficult for the parents, many of whom quite naturally struggle with hearing their baby cry in the night, but resist the temptation to intervene, so allowing the child to "self-soothe" and learn to reinitiate sleep by themselves, the so-called "controlled crying" approach. Some cannot stand the sound of their child crying at night and continue to intervene, but pay the price of having their own sleep disturbed for much longer (sometimes several years longer) than those who implement the controlled crying approaches.

This is a contentious area, with two clear camps either endorsing the approach, or remaining staunchly against it on the grounds that it is cruel to the child to let them cry during the night. Leaving a child to cry uncontrollably for a long period of time is neglectful and should never be advised. However, attending immediately to a child every time they wake up during the night becomes a self-fulfilling prophecy, the child gets more and more used to the attention, and will resist more (and for longer) should that attention begin to be reduced; which is ultimately what every parent desires in order to regain full nights of unbroken sleep. So the attention needs to be reduced eventually, and the sooner that a child learns to sleep through the night by themselves (after the age of six months or so in healthy, full-term children), then the better for everyone.

As with all aspects of parenting, there is no manual, and each family needs to approach the issue of their child's sleep in their own way. There are grades of strategies, from co-sleeping, continual attention, and immediate intervention approaches, through to extinction strategies at the other end of the spectrum. Neither of these are particularly ideal and there is a middle ground, gradual extinction, which most parents adopt, either by active choice, or by working it out naturalistically, on the hoof. These approaches will be described in the following sections.

Co-sleeping, continual attention, immediate intervention

Sleeping with a very small child in the same bed as her parent(s) is never a good idea, and is actively recommended against by midwives and paediatricians. The reason being that every year several children are suffocated by their (very tired) parents rolling on top of them during the night. From a less serious perspective, co-sleeping is not recommended as the child and parent(s) disturb each other during the night with noise and movements.

Having the child in a crib or Moses basket next to the parent's bed is recommended up to around the first six-to-twelve months of life (for healthy children) to enable the parent(s) to intervene with feeding and resettling as required by the child. Thereafter it is usually beneficial for both the child and others in the house to move the child to their own room if possible, where noise and movements during the night are less likely to disturb all parties. Co-sleeping approaches tend to benefit the child, but not the parents in terms of sleep.

Extinction approaches

At the other end of the spectrum is that of extinction, whereby once the parent(s) are confident that their child is: (1) tired and ready for bed; (2) clean; and (3) fed, that the child is put down to sleep whilst they are still awake, but sleepy. The parent(s) then leave the child to go to sleep by themselves. If the child is awake during the night, and the parent(s) are confident that the child is still clean and not requiring another feed, then the child is ignored until he goes back to sleep by themselves. Obviously if their child is very distressed and crying for a long time then some intervention may well be required. This approach tends to favour the parents rather than the child in terms of sleep *in the short term*, but in the longer term the child learns to initiate, maintain, and reinitiate sleep by themselves.

This autonomy in sleep is an important developmental milestone for the child, and also helps others in the house to have and maintain undisturbed and restful sleep. However, some parents simply cannot bear to hear their child crying and feel that they must intervene. Criticism of this approach has been vigorous and widespread, with claims that leaving a crying child raises their cortisol levels and can lead to anxiety in the child. This may well be the case for children who are neglected for long periods, but this approach, if administered appropriately can encourage a child to sleep through the night after a few weeks, which is arguably less stressful for the child and the parent(s) who continue to arise to attend to their child multiple times per night for several years. So these two, polarised approaches both have problems which has given rise to the middle ground approach that is gradual, or graded extinction.

Gradual extinction

Extinction is a psychological term for removing a behaviour completely and immediately. Such approaches tend to "hurt", but achieve results quickly if maintained and adhered to. A good example of this is giving up smoking, one can just stop, and then never start again. Initially this is very hard, but after a few weeks the problem is resolved. Many people struggle with this, and instead opt for a more graded approach, gradually cutting down, perhaps moving to a brand of cigarettes with a lower nicotine content. This hurts less, but takes longer. Similarly, with child sleep, the graded approach is less stressful for the parent(s) and child, but can take longer. The process works by gradually reducing the amount of intervention, and increasing the wait time to intervene, with a child who wakes in the night. Gradually reducing contact and minimising interventions with less-and-less time and attention given to the child who has woken during the night. There are many different models, but an example is given below in Figure 22 as a guideline that will need tailoring to the individuals' needs and the proclivities of the family.

Over time this approach is very effective, but does require tailoring to the sensibilities of the parents, as well as to the needs of the child, especially if the child is unwell or has specific medical needs requiring intervention during the night.

Graded extinction has emerged as the most favourable approach for parents to adopt for use with their children's sleep, and these approaches tend to be most effective for younger children who have not had the time to habituate to less effective sleep practices. In healthy youngsters, learning to sleep by themselves is usually possible from around six to eight months of age, and can often be introduced and implemented effectively within a couple of weeks for children of six to eight months of age. For older children this can take longer to introduce and implement successfully as, generally speaking, the child has had more parental attention during the night-time and has habituated to getting this attention. The removal of this attention can therefore be more stressful for the older child. So the golden rule is to try and begin this as early as possible (after around six months of age), and the faster one can get through, what is a difficult and challenging experience, then the better for everyone.

- Leave the child for five minutes to get to sleep by themselves, if they are quietening then try and leave this for longer. Then resettle if required. Try and then leave the child for longer the next time, around seven minutes, and then longer again on the third occasion, maybe for ten minutes. When intervening, try to avoid talking to, moving/touching the child, so they get used to a reduction in the amount of attention that they receive during the night-time.
- Adopt a similar approach for night-time awakenings.
- Increase times as the days and weeks go by, leaving the child for longer and longer, and minimising physical and verbal contact with the child during the night.
- Give lots of love and attention during the daytime, when it is appropriate to have action, and save the night-time for inaction.

Figure 22. An example of a gradual extinction approach.

This is a contentious issue and, as a result, graded extinction is the recommended practice, with each family deciding upon a model which they are as comfortable with as possible. Finally, in terms of the treatment of sleeping problems in children, the major consideration is the age of the child and their requirements for both night-time and daytime sleep.

Sleep and age considerations

There are no absolutes for sleep, as people can be either long sleepers or short sleepers at any age, and infants may have more or less of a requirement for sleep during the day and night-time. As a rough guide Table 5 below shows approximate night-time and daytime sleep requirements for children at different ages.

These data are only approximated as each child will differ in their own specific requirements. No one will know better than the child's main carer(s) how much sleep their child will need if they have sensible and realistic ideas about sleep. However, there is always opportunity to meet a parent who believes that eight hours of sleep per night is enough for their three-year-old!

Table 5. Approximate sleep and nap requirements for children at different ages.

Age	Sleep requirement during the night	Number of daytime naps	Average duration of each daytime nap
1 month	Variable	Variable	Variable
6 months	9–11	3–4	30–45 minutes
1 year	9–11	2–3	30–45 minutes
2 years	10–11	1–2	45–90 minutes
3 years	10–12	0–1	30–60 minutes
5 years	9–11	0	–
8 years	8–10	0	–
10 years	8–10	0	–
15 years	7–9	0	–
18 years	6–9	0	–

CONSIDERATIONS FOR VULNERABLE GROUPS   139

Recently a mnemonic was published to aid in organising the common recommendations for managing sleep in children, the "ABCs of SLEEPING" (Allen, Howlett, Coulombe, & Corkum, 2015):

1. Age appropriate Bedtimes and wake-times with Consistency.
2. Schedules and routines.
3. Location.
4. Exercise and diet.
5. no Electronics in the bedroom or before bed.
6. Positivity.
7. Independence when falling asleep.
8. Needs of child met during the day.
9. equals Great sleep.

These recommendations emphasise the importance of consistent routines both during the daytime and the night-time, that sleep is encouraged to be initiated and maintained without the intervention of an adult carer and that this is conducted in a consistent place (i.e., the child's own bedroom). Sleep hygiene elements enter these recommendations in terms of avoiding the use of electronic screens at and around bedtime; and ensuring that the child is supported in their physical and emotional needs, placing a key emphasis on positivity and loving care and attention.

Teenagers

As children get older their requirements for sleep change in a physiological sense, but their developing social lives enforce changes in their routine as they begin to make more and more decisions for themselves. The reduced requirement for sleep as we go through the teenage years is offset by changing physiological changes resulting from puberty and growth spurts, which may, at times, increase the requirement for more sleep than usual. Reductions in sleep time also tend to be driven by normal sociological changes associated with wanting to be more "grown-up" and to opt for later and later bedtimes, like their parents and older friends. The reduced academic performance and increased negative behaviours associated with sleep-deprived children is well documented, but it is often a challenge for parents to encourage their teenager to get the amount of sleep that they require as:

1. Teenagers do not want to go to bed early anymore.
2. They do not want to be told to go to bed early anymore.
3. They do not tend to listen when they are asked to go to bed early.
4. Teens do not want to get up in the morning.
5. They have to get up at a reasonable hour, because they need to go to school.

Hence, many teenagers lock themselves away in their bedrooms, stay up late playing computer games/social networking on the internet etc. and then have to get up in enough time to get to school. As a result, there is widespread sleep deprivation in this group, which is of concern for behaviour management at school and at home, as well as a concern about academic achievement potential. There is an emerging body of research examining later school start times for adolescents which has shown promising initial results in terms of improved behaviour and psychological outcomes for delayed school start times on the performance of teenagers, but rigorous trials are still required to confirm these promising initial results (Minges & Redeker, 2016).

As with most things, getting in early solves a bigger problem later on down the line, so if one has children who sleep well and enjoy their sleep, then these are more likely to "graduate" through the teenage years and into adulthood with resilient, refreshing, and enjoyable sleep. Others with a propensity for disturbed sleep, or whom are distressed or traumatised in some way, may likely experience problems with their sleep, and adolescence is a stressful time.

Fostering a strong relationship that is trusting and enables good quality, bidirectional communication between the teenager and their parent(s) or carers is the best way to proceed with encouraging them to take enough sleep and at reasonable times. Children need to develop autonomy in their decision-making as they get older and deciding when, where, and how to sleep is something that we all do as adults, and something that we are all quite particular about regardless of the quality of our sleep. Young children are taught how, when, and where to sleep by their parents and at some stage during their teenage years, these decisions quite naturally pass from the parent to the young adult. The transition is usually rocky and by no means specific to just sleep, many other aspects of life's choices and decisions are "handed over" to the young adult during this time. Good quality communication, and an ability to successfully discuss and negotiate, is essential to assist smooth transitions such as sleep-related decisions through this time.

So far in this chapter we have explored sleep changes across the human lifespan and identified some considerations and age-specific treatment approaches, there are however a multitude of conditions that the practicing healthcare professional may encounter in their daily work, some of which have specific impacts on sleep, and may require specific considerations for the treatment of sleep problems. Therefore, the remainder of this chapter will describe some of the issues relating to sleep in various groups of people with commonly presenting conditions, and some additional considerations for their treatment.

People living with chronic pain

Pain is extremely common with millions of people living with pain as part of their daily lives. The experience of living with chronic pain has a twofold impact on sleep. First, and most obviously, the pain itself causes discomfort and this inability to obtain, and to maintain, a comfortable position in bed often makes sleep difficult to initiate and to maintain undisturbed. Furthermore, turning over, or otherwise moving, during sleep can result in pressure or movement that causes pain and this in turn wakes the individual from their sleep. Second, is the distress and anxiety of managing a life with chronic pain, and these psychological sequelae can also impact negatively on sleep. There are therefore two additional directions over and above the usual REST principles, in which one can then approach the management and treatment of sleep problems for this group of people: (1) Managing the pain with analgesia, pillows/supports, orthopaedic beds etc.; and (2) working psychologically with the depression, anxiety, trauma etc. which may be associated with the individual's pain.

Cognitive behavioural therapy for insomnia has been shown to be effective for the management of sleep problems in people living with chronic pain (Tang, 2009, Finan, Buenaver, Coryell, & Smith, 2014), as has co-therapy (CBT for pain and insomnia, delivered concurrently) (Pigeon et al., 2012). Usually people living with conditions that cause chronic pain are under the care of another treating professional (or professionals), often including: anaesthesiologists, physiotherapists, occupational therapists, psychologists, and/or nurses. As such it is essential to work collaboratively with these other treating professionals;

contacting them at the outset of treatment is most important in order to make sure that any treatments provided are synchronous and complimentary to those already being provided by these other professionals.

In terms of interventions from the REST programme, it is important to role these out at a carefully defined pace, and one that is in keeping with the capacity of the individual client, especially with respect to: (1) their functional capacity; (2) their ability to engage with interventions around feelings of fatigue (including timing and duration); (3) their commitments to other therapeutic interventions (e.g., physiotherapy); (4) their experiences of consuming medications (which may have an impact on their capacity to engage (both physically and cognitively)); and (5) their levels of fatigue. Often the initial psychoeducation elements of REST, especially that of the phenomenon, function, and impact of the circadian rhythm can be particularly effective for these clients.

Chronic fatigue syndrome (CFS), fibromyalgia, and myalgic encephalomyelitis (ME)

Disturbed sleep in CFS, fibromyalgia, and ME is almost universally experienced by those living with these conditions. Common manifestations of CFS, fibromyalgia, and ME are those of prolonged resting, inactivity, and sometimes napping behaviours during the day time. As we saw in Chapter Two, the practice of over sleeping (hypersomnia) is associated with feelings that are similar in nature to insomnia, that is, paradoxically feeling tired, lethargic, and unrested. As a result, those with CFS, fibromyalgia, and ME, although perhaps needing to rest for certain periods during the day, may be experiencing the symptoms of hypersomnia if they are engaging in napping, or sleeping for excessively long periods through the night. Resting and pacing of activities has been recommended as a treatment of choice for people living with these conditions, to better enable them to manage the symptoms of their illness and improve functionality (Bested & Marshall, 2015). If rest is required during the daytime, then it is recommended that this rest be taken in a room other than the bedroom and that sleep is avoided at such times. Furthermore, if possible, a reduction to pre-morbid sleep times should be considered if the client is sleeping excessively during the night, in an attempt to avoid any symptoms of hypersomnia. This, coupled with gradual increases in scheduled daytime activity (preferably outside under conditions of natural sunlight) may well serve to improve the debilitating symptoms experienced by people living with CFS, fibromyalgia, and ME.

There is a noticeable lack of research on sleep treatment in these groups, and much work is required to be conducted in this area before any firm conclusions can be drawn about the efficacy of such treatments; other than those that have been reported by anecdote and the experience of those applying these techniques with such clients. That said it is certainly worth trying some of the behavioural and psychological approaches detailed above and in Chapter Five, just with sensitive attenuation to the pace and capacity of the clients themselves as we saw in the previous section on those living with chronic pain.

Multiple sclerosis

Sleep disturbances and chronic fatigue in people with multiple sclerosis (MS) are very common presentations affecting up to seventy-five per cent of people with the condition (Bakshi et al., 2000). Although there is a lack of research on both the pharmacological and psychological/ behavioural treatment of fatigue and sleep disturbances in MS (Lee, Newell, Ziegler, & Topping, 2008). Some recent findings have shown good results for the use of CBTi in people with MS, all be it in a relatively small sample of only fifteen cases (Clancy, Drerup, & Sullivan, 2015), and CBTi has been specifically recommended for use in the management of sleep disturbances in people with MS (Baron, Corden, Jin, & Mohr, 2011).

Similarly, as with people experiencing CFS, fibromyalgia, and ME (in the section above), there may well be a propensity for hypersomnia in people with MS, and the curtailment of sleep duration may be a useful treatment strategy for those people with MS who are sleeping for long periods of time, alongside the careful pacing of activity and scheduling of rest periods. However, sleep and fatigue issues in MS may well be complicated by the underlying neurological changes seen in MS, as well as the different types of the disease. The more aggressive, primary progressive form of MS have increased impact on sleep and fatigue than the less insidious, relapsing/remitting forms (Lee, Newell, Ziegler, & Topping, 2008).

There is a possibility here that the pathogenesis and progression of the various forms of MS are suggestive of different underlying neural correlates, which would potentially inform different treatment strategies for the management of fatigue and sleep disturbance in the different subtypes of MS, but this remains to be fully explored and explained. With regard to REST interventions for this group, then a similar approach to working with people living with chronic pain, fibromyalgia, ME, and CFS (as in the previous two sections) is recommended.

Alcohol dependency syndrome

Alcohol is the most common self-prescribed hypnotic agent in the developed world. Millions of people use alcohol to help them to get to sleep every night. Alcohol certainly has soporific effects, which is why people often turn to it to help them to get to sleep. There are, however, a number of problems with the use (or abuse) of alcohol in this way. First, alcohol alters the sleep architecture, reducing the amount of slow wave sleep and increasing the amount of REM sleep (Lands, 1999). As a result, people who have consumed moderate to large amounts of alcohol in the evening before going to bed experience sleep that is non-refreshing and that has potentially not effectively encoded and consolidated memories into the individuals' schematic neural pathways (from the end of Chapter One). This leads to mood consequences that are likely to exacerbate more alcohol seeking behaviours the next day. Second, alcohol is a toxin that requires elimination from the system. This elimination requires a lot of water and as a result an intoxicated individual will often wake early in the morning feeling dehydrated and needing to take on more water. Dehydration is a cause of early morning awakening (EMA), which is one form of insomnia (from Chapter Two) and this is very common in people with alcohol dependency syndrome. Finally, alcohol is addictive and people that begin to use alcohol regularly can easily cross a threshold into abusing the substance, which can then have increased impact on poor sleep and mood, thus having an insidious, circular effect on an individual.

A review of CBTi treatments for insomnia co-morbid with alcohol dependency published in 2014 showed a small number of studies examining the efficacy of psychobehavioural approaches for the treatment and management of insomnia in this group. Although the numbers of available studies are small, initial findings indicate the utility of cognitive and behavioural approaches in the successful treatment of insomnia in those who are chronic users of alcohol (Brooks & Wallen, 2014). It is worth noting here that recovery from alcohol can take a considerable amount of time, with sleep disturbances persisting sometimes for a long time after abstinence. These persisting sleep problems can promote relapse and so a person with alcohol dependency syndrome with concomitant sleep problems will often require significant amounts of support for protracted time periods whilst they are in recovery.

When implementing the interventions described in the REST programme for people who are dependent or recovering from alcohol it is again imperative to work collaboratively with any other treating professional(s), to consider the pacing of delivery as in the previous conditions above in sections D, E , and F of this chapter. Particular attention should be given to the client's memory, due to the potential amnestic effects of alcohol, and to the potential for relapse in both sleep experiences and drinking behaviours during what can often be a protracted period of recovery.

Eating disorders

Sleep-related eating disorder is classified as a parasomnia, where eating during the night occurs as a complex somnambulism and is usually beyond the awareness of the individual at the time of the behavioural occurrence. This should not be confused with nocturnal eating syndrome, which is characterised as an eating disorder that is often associated with insomnia, where an individual will have awareness of eating at the time of the behaviour (Auger, 2006). There is little published information on the sleep of those with eating disorders and therefore any treatment options remain relatively unexplored and certainly under-researched.

For sleep-related eating disorders (the parasomnia), then CBTi methods detailed above in Chapters Four and Five are worthy of implementation, in order to minimise the impact and subsequent effects of the parasomnia. For the condition of nocturnal eating syndrome, then a co-treatment of CBTi and psychotherapy for eating disorders is warranted. A carefully conducted differential diagnosis between the two conditions is initially required in order to direct the client to the most appropriate form of treatment. Awareness of the behaviour is the key to delineating which condition is being experienced, if the client is aware of their eating behaviours then this is likely to be a nocturnal eating syndrome requiring co-treatment with CBTi and psychotherapeutic intervention for eating disorder. Otherwise, where the client is unaware of their nocturnal eating behaviours, then it is likely that are experiencing a parasomnia, whereby REST interventions may suffice in isolation.

Head injury

Sleep disturbances are very common after brain injury (Ouellet, Beaulieu-Bonneau, & Morin, 2015), but again there is little research evidence detailing the sleep experiences and certainly the treatment of sleeping problems in these people. Available data suggests that sleep outcomes in the immediate aftermath of a closed head brain injury are better predictors of outcome than the Glasgow Coma Scale score, with those showing EEG measured response profiles and less aberrant sleep architecture (sleep staging and shifts between stages) having better survival and rehabilitation trajectories than those showing less response and more disturbance to their sleep architecture (Evans & Bartlett, 1995). There is also evidence of increased awakenings during the night in people who have sustained closed head injuries that is associated with negative behavioural manifestations during the day (Prigatano, Stahl, Orr, & Zeiner, 1982). These are also associated with negative consequences for carers, both during the night-time and during the daytime; and in terms of management of the person they are caring for as well as themselves and commitments to other family members etc. The impact on carers is discussed below in the "Carers" section of this Chapter.

In terms of treatment of sleeping problems in those who have sustained a closed head injury it is worth noting that (similarly to people who have experienced a stroke—see below in Section J of this chapter) it is not uncommon for people who have sustained a closed head injury to sleep for lengthy periods in the immediate aftermath of the index accident (Ouellet, Beaulieu-Bonneau, & Morin, 2015), and that this extended sleep may well occur for a number of months following the injury, dependent on a number of factors shown in Figure 23 below:

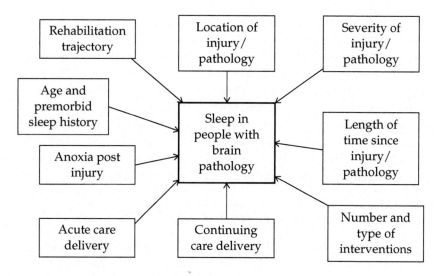

Figure 23. Factors which may affect the sleep of someone who has experienced brain pathology.

As a result of the complexity of brain pathology, the impact on sleep may be mild to severe depending on the number and extent of the influence of those factors presented in Figure 23 above. As such, it is imperative in the management and treatment of sleep problems in this group of people to collect a good history, which enquires of these factors in order to ascertain which elements may be fixed, and which are perhaps more malleable in the management of the sleep of such an individual. Of note here is the consideration again of the "two-year" rule that we saw in the section titled "Hypersomnia" in Chapter Two , that often people with brain injury may still be experiencing brain healing up to two years after the index accident; and so interventions may well need to consider this prolonged period of brain healing in terms of the level and pace of delivery of any planned interventions (Ruttan, Martin, Liu, Colella, & Green, 2008; Schretlen & Shapiro 2003).

There is a lack of well-defined research studies in the area of sleep management in people who have sustained brain injuries, although there has been suggestion that psychobehavioural sleep interventions have merit for this group (Ouellet & Morin, 2004; Ouellet,

Beaulieu-Bonneau, & Morin, 2015). This is complex and challenging for the treating healthcare professional and is by no means limited to sleep management, many other aspects of a head injured client will be affected by their index accident and by the treatment and experiences they have received, and lived with, since their sustained injuries (Bassetti, 2005). Careful pacing and close collaboration with often a large number other treating healthcare and legal professionals is essential for the effective management of sleep disturbances in this group of clients. If these are well managed, then interventions from REST can prove very successful in the management of sleep disturbances in this client group.

Autism spectrum disorder (ASD)

There is also a paucity of research available on the sleep of people who are living on the autistic spectrum, although that which is available does indicate that children with ASD sleep less well than those children without the condition; on both subjectively and objectively reported outcomes (Souders et al., 2009). Children with ASD have also been reported to have more problems with initiating their sleep and have an increased number of night-time awakenings than typically developing children (Krakowiak, Goodlin-Jones, Hertz-Picciotto, Croen, & Hansen, 2008). A reduced amount of REM sleep has also been reported in children with ASD compared with typically developing children (Williams-Buckley et al., 2010).

With regard to treatment strategies for sleep problems in children with ASD melatonin has shown promise in a few studies at increasing total sleep time and reducing sleep latency (Wirojanan et al., 2009). However, there is a lack of large, well-designed studies examining the efficacy of melatonin (including the dosage and timing of administration). Therefore, the utility of melatonin in the management of sleep problems in this group remains to be fully explored (Guénolé, et al., 2011). Behavioural interventions for improving sleep in children with ASD have centred on exercise and parent-education programmes, both of which have shown positive effects on the sleep outcomes of children with ASD, although these studies are very few in number and much more work is required in this area to draw firm conclusions about their efficacy. Indeed, very few studies are available in the area of sleep in ASD with one recent review of behavioural interventions in ASD failing to find any (Weaver, 2015). At the time of writing there was no literature available to report on regarding the sleep and treatment of sleep disturbances in adults on the ASD spectrum.

As a result of this lack of research in the field of assessment and treatment of sleep problems in people with ASD some caution is required in the delivery of any form of intervention, without a sound knowledge-base to which to refer. As such, a careful and thorough assessment is required involving the person with ASD (taking into account the capacity of the person to engage and comply with any suggested interventions), their family/carers and other treating professionals. This is essential in order to design appropriately paced interventions that are person-centred, sensitive to family situations, and which takes into consideration the number and type of other interventions that are in place. Of particular note here is the phenomenon of hyperactivity in some children with ASD which is a common behavioural manifestation in this group of clients. Excessive levels of daytime activity can lead to excessive tiredness and this can then have a negative impact on behaviour and mood. Sometimes attention to the reduction of daytime activity is warranted through the scheduling of rest-periods, or attenuating periods of activity so that the client is not excessively active for long periods.

People with dementia

There is a fairly large body of work that has reported on the sleep of people with dementia and this can usefully be divided into the three most common causes of dementia namely: Alzheimer's disease, vascular dementia, and the Lewy body dementias.

Alzheimer's disease

The deposited Tau protein plaques, which characterise the development and progression of Alzheimer's disease, choke and interfere with nerve transmissions throughout the brain in a gradual and irreversible way. As the disease progresses very often there are changes experienced to sleep (Bliwise, 1993). These are known to exacerbate other symptoms (e.g., behavioural manifestations such as nocturnal wandering) (Klein et al., 1999) and accelerate the rate of cognitive decline (Lee & Thomas, 2011), as well as posing a significant challenge for carers who have their own sleep disturbed by the person they are caring for, especially if they wander the house during the night (Livingston, Manela, & Katona, 1996). Not everyone with dementia experiences poor sleep, and it may well be the case that those who continue to sleep well with their advancing dementia may do so because they have always had resilient sleep.

Vascular dementia

Stroke-related neurodegeneration progresses in a step-wise manner unlike the gradual deterioration in brain function associated with Alzheimer's disease. These step-wise reductions in capacity are associated with ischaemic events in the brain. In other words, when an individual has a stroke, then there is an immediate loss of function which may then "heal" to a certain extent after the event, but some loss of function remains, as a result of scar tissue and neuronal damage within the brain. Furthermore, the loss of function that is experienced is very much dependent on the location of the lesion(s) and the severity of the stroke itself. In the immediate aftermath of a stroke it is not uncommon for an individual to sleep for much longer periods of time as the lesion heals within the brain, similarly to those who have sustained a brain injury. If lesions are experienced in the region of those areas which are important for the regulation and control of sleep then much sleep disturbance can be seen following a stroke (Alberti, 2014; Bassetti, 2005) but, again, this is highly dependent on the location and severity of the stroke as well as other factors presented above in Figure 23.

Lewy body dementias

There are two forms of Lewy body dementia and they form the two ends of a spectrum, with Parkinson's disease dementia at one end and dementia with Lewy bodies at the other. Parkinson's disease (PD) is associated with balance and gait problems, tremor and other "autonomic" problems such as temperature regulation, memory problems. Other behavioural manifestations associated with dementia tend to occur in the latter stages of the disease. Dementia with Lewy bodies (DLB), although sharing a pathogenic mechanism with PD is somewhat different, with dementia symptoms occurring earlier in the disease course and the experience of (usually) vivid visual hallucinations, but with less of the balance and gait issues that are common with people with PD. The pathogenic mechanism for both of these forms of dementia is the deposition of alpha-synuclein protein (unlike Tau protein in Alzheimer's disease) and these tend to clump into inclusion-like bundles, interfering with nerve transmission, but not choking neurons in the same way as Tau in Alzheimer's disease (Boeve, Silber, & Ferman, 2004).

As with vascular dementia, the location of these inclusions determines the functions that become most affected, but these inclusions can be quite diffusely spread around the brain and brainstem. One very common manifestation of both of these Lewy body dementias is that of REM sleep behaviour disorder (RBD). The symptom of RBD is so common in people with PD and DLB that it is a core diagnostic feature of these conditions. RBD is associated with a loss of REM sleep atonia, in that people who have the symptom no longer remain paralysed during periods of REM sleep and can act out their dreams (sometimes quite violently). RBD has also been noted to occasionally be prodromal for the development of DLB and PD with some individuals reported to experience RBD up to fourteen years before developing PD or DLB (Boeve, Silber, & Ferman, 2004).

Sleep management in dementia

This is a complex and challenging area for the healthcare professional, or family member caring for someone with dementia, as well as for the person themselves. Poor sleep is very common across all forms of dementia, but not necessarily universal, some people, even with quite advanced stages of dementia can still sleep relatively well, and this may well be because they always slept well (thinking back to Spielman's predisposing factors from Chapter Two.) Others, who may not have always slept so well, often experience disturbed sleep and napping behaviours during the daytime. These napping behaviours have been shown to be protective of the rate of cognitive decline in people with Alzheimer's disease if regularly napping for an hour or less during the day, but the opposite has been found for those sleeping for more than an hour and especially those sleeping for two or more hours during the day, that is, these people have an accelerated rate of cognitive decline compared with those who do not habitually nap (Asada, Motonaga, Yamagata, Uno, & Takahashi, 2000).

The training of healthcare professionals in the management of sleep disturbances in dementia is scant and has been identified as a priority for treating professionals, especially in light of the high prevalence of sleep problems in dementia, the increased demand on family carers, the impact of sleep disturbance on the progression of dementia and the increasing numbers of older people in society (Lee & Thomas, 2011).

Traditionally sleep disturbances in dementia have been managed with sedative/hypnotic medications, but, due to the high levels of adverse events associated with these medications in people with dementia, nonpharmacological methods have been recommended, including: sleep hygiene, CBTi, and bright light therapy (including melatonin) (David et al., 2010; Guarnieri & Sorbi, 2015). There has been some promising research with bright light therapy in the management of sleep in dementia (Van Someren, Kessler, Mirmiran, & Swaab, 1997) and melatonin (de Jonghe, Korevaar, van Munster, & de Rooij, 2010). Although there is a paucity of research on other psychobehavioural treatment interventions for older people with dementia, as well as criticism as to the lack of training that clinicians receive in the management of sleep disturbances in dementia and the sensitivity of instruments, such as the DSM-V, to specifically diagnose and guide treatment interventions for this client group (Lee & Thomas, 2011).

Interventions from the REST programme as well as other psychobehavioural interventions (such as bright light therapy as detailed above) are worthy of consideration for this group of clients. However, it is again important to: ensure careful pacing; consideration of the physical and cognitive capacity of the client, collaboration with family members/carers, and to interact closely with other treating healthcare professionals and the other interventions and medications the client may be prescribed with.

Carers

Anyone who provides care for another person is likely to have their sleep disturbed from two separate, but inextricably linked directions. First, the direct impact of the person they provide care for who may be rising in the night and disturbing their carers sleep, and second, from the anxiety and distress that is often associated with a demanding caring role.

Sometimes caring confers pleasure and reward, especially in the domain of new parenting, but other forms of caring are usually associated with at least some level of distress, especially when providing care for someone who has sustained a brain injury or an older person who is living with dementia (Livingston, Manela, & Katona, 1996). This stress may be exacerbated even more so when the carer themselves is an older person, potentially having their own physical and/or mental health issues. Carer stress has also been reported to be increased in those providing care for people with Parkinson's Disease Dementia and Dementia with Lewy Bodies, compared with those caring for people with Alzheimer's disease and vascular dementia, exacerbated by the presence of cognitive fluctuations, psychotic manifestations (such as hallucinations), and mood disturbances (Lee, McKeith, Mosimann, Ghosh-Nodyal, & Thomas, 2013). This carer stress can accelerate the breakdown of family, community-based care provision and precipitate a move of the person with dementia to an institutional care setting (Kesselring et al., 2001, Thommessen et al., 2002). Although this can be ameliorated by supporting carers with respite care provision, which has been shown to reduce carer stress (Lee, Morgan, & Lindesay, 2004), and improve carers' sleep (Lee, Morgan, & Lindesay, 2007).

Unfortunately, very little research has been conducted on the psychobehavioural treatment of sleep problems in carers, only one study, with a very small sample of just ten participants, has shown some positive effects on carer sleep with the use of meditation and imagery training (Jain, Nazarian, & Lavretsky, 2014).

Owing to the effectiveness of psychobehavioural interventions for the management of sleep in adults and older people generally, then there is no reason to assume that interventions and advice from the REST programme would not benefit this client group too. However, extra considerations are required for carers in terms of the management of their daytime activity based around their caring roles. Pacing daytime activity, scheduling rest during the daytime, attention to bed and waking routines, and managing any distress associated with the caring role can be especially important for this client group, often requiring collaboration with other family members, treating healthcare professionals and potentially scheduling periods of respite from the caring role (be those *ad hoc*, short-term assistance at home, or scheduled periods of booked respite care in a local hospital for the person being cared for).

Pregnancy

Sleep disturbances during normal, healthy pregnancies are frequently reported, with pregnant women often describing difficulty falling asleep, frequent nocturnal awakenings, and an increased incidence of sleep disordered breathing and snoring (Mindell & Jacobson, 2000).

A fuller description of sleep in pregnancy is described in Chapter Seven of John Wilks's book: *Choices in Pregnancy and Childbirth* (Lee, 2015.) To summarise here: there is a lack of evidence on sleep in the first trimester, but one study has reported an increased total sleep time during this time (Hedman, Pohjasvaara, Tolonen, Suhonen-Malm, & Myllylä, 2002), although another study has reported no change in total sleep time in the first, second, or even third trimesters (Little, McNamara, & Miller, 2014).

The more prominent changes in sleep are reported for the second and, particularly, the third trimesters. As pregnancy progresses into the second trimester time spent awake during the night has been reported to increase significantly (Hertz et al., 1992), from approximately thirty-five minutes per night in the first trimester, to around forty-five minutes in the second trimester and up to one hour in the third. These increases in nocturnal wakefulness are seen in tandem with increases in the number of nocturnal awakenings as women progress through the stages of their pregnancies (Little, McNamara, & Miller, 2014). The amount of slow wave sleep has also been reported to diminish through the course of a normal pregnancy (Wilson et al., 2011) along with reports of increased napping behaviours (Mindell & Jacobson, 2000). These measured changes mirror those that are reported subjectively by women as they advance with pregnancy, with fatigue, tiredness, and sleep disturbances being common, to the point of being normal features of pregnancy. Sometimes though, these feelings can have a detrimental impact on the mother's mood. Tikotzky & Sadeh (2009) reported significant links between the mother's cognitions during pregnancy and the sleep of their infants once born. There is also evidence of sleep disturbance in mothers during and after pregnancy, which can impact negatively on the relationship between the mother and her child (Chang, Pien, Duntley, & Macones, 2010; Pires, Andersen, Giovernardi, & Tufik, 2010).

The management of sleep disturbances in pregnancy has received next to no research attention, with no studies available to refer to for interventions that might be efficacious for pregnant women to improve their sleep. There is also no research available for new fathers either. Anecdotal reports suggest that the more support that new parents have around them, to aid with their sleep, during the latter stages of pregnancy for the mother, and post-partum for both parents then the better they feel. It is important for parents to work as a team, supporting each other with rest and sleep when, and wherever, possible. The first few months are challenging in this respect for every new parent (as above in the section about younger children in this chapter) and sleeping in shifts is a good way to help everyone to get through this time unfazed. An example is presented below in Figure 24.

In this way, hopefully, the mother will get undisturbed sleep from 9pm to around 2am (about five hours), which provides her with those first three circadian cycles of sleep which have a large proportion of deep, slow wave sleep (from Chapter One), and then more disturbed sleep from 3am through to the end of the night (although this is lighter and less restorative sleep). And, again, hopefully, the father will get around seven hours of undisturbed sleep from midnight through to 7am.

This is all well and good for families with healthy children, but for those who are single parents, and/or those with poorly children this can be an exceptional challenge. The only answer is: ENLIST HELP and enlist it from wherever it is safely and practically available. Sleep where

---

- Mother sleeps during the day, when baby sleeps, although this may only be light sleep if the child does not sleep for long periods.
- In the evening the child is fed and put down to sleep around 7–8pm, then mother gets to bed around 9pm.
- Father then feeds the child in the late evening around 10–11pm, before going to bed.
- Mother then rises during the night to feed at around 2–3am, and again around 5–6am.
- All rise around 7am.

Figure 24. An example of shift-sleeping for new parenting.

and when you can to provide the energy needed for childcare, and it requires lots!

The menopause

Sleep changes as we age in both men and women, but the menopause is associated with additional changes to sleep that are likely influenced by changes (reductions) in the secretion of the female gonadotrophic hormones, oestrogen and progesterone. Peri-menopausal women have been shown to have reduced slow wave sleep and increased sleep latencies than women who are not experiencing the menopause; and that these women sleep objectively worse than age-matched men (Bixler et al., 2009). These findings are congruent with both objective and self-reported poor sleep of women who are experiencing the menopause compared with pre- and post-menopausal women (Young, Rabago, Zgierska, Austin, & Finn, 2003).

One of the most common complaints during the time of the menopause (and that which often causes discomfort during the night) is that of the phenomenon of "hot flashes". Most menopausal women whom experience severe hot flashes report poor sleep, with around forty per cent reaching the clinical criteria for insomnia (Joffe, Massler, & Sharkey, 2010). Managing the temperature of the bedroom by adjusting heating and ventilation, and also the weight of bedding, has the potential to ameliorate the intrusion of these on sleep and should be considered as a possible intervention for improving sleep around this time, although research is unfortunately lacking in this area. Interestingly, the use of hormone replacement therapy (HRT), which has strong support in alleviating many of the negative symptoms of the menopause, has also shown a positive impact on sleep. With women on HRT programmes showing improved sleep outcomes than those menopausal women not in such programmes (Bixler et al., 2009). Although no psychobehavioural intervention studies for the management of sleep disturbances in menopausal women have been conducted to date, they have been put forward as a potentially useful treatment for insomnia in this group (Joffe, Massler, & Sharkey, 2010).

Sleep in recreational drug users

There is not a large body of research into the sleep experienced by those whom consume recreational drugs, however there is evidence of a significant impact to the sleep architecture as a result of consuming pretty much the whole range of recreational drugs. Including: heroin; methadone; the other opiates; cocaine; MDMA (ecstasy); amphetamines; and cannabis (marijuana). Cocaine, amphetamines, and MDMA have been shown to increase nocturnal wakefulness, increase arousal, and suppress REM sleep, and these changes can persist in heavy users during periods of abstinence. Acute cannabis consumption has been reported to increase SWS, although reductions in SWS can also be seen, as well as reducing the amount of REM sleep. Difficulty initiating sleep and the occurrence of disturbing dreams has also been reported on withdrawal (Schierenbeck, Riemann, Berger, & Hornyak, 2008). Heroin and methadone use has been shown to reduce REM sleep and stage two sleep, with rebounds in REM sleep and SWS on seen withdrawal. There are also significant impairments to perception, learning, and memory in people abusing the opiate drugs (Chester, 1985).

With regard to the treatment of sleep problems in this group the situation is complicated by the pharmacokinetic effects of these drugs on the sleep architecture that is unlikely to be resolved psychobehaviourally whilst these agents are still being consumed. As a result, the effective treatment of a sleep problem in this group requires the abstinence of the client from their drug consumption; and this precipitates a further challenge for the clinician in managing their client's substance withdrawal. There are also, very often, underlying psychological issues with such clients, which may have had an influence on their history of drug taking; and also a high prevalence of polypharmacy, with many drug users consuming a range of substances, further complicating the work of the clinician. Added to this are the often protracted time periods required in abstinence for "normal" sleep architecture to resume, sometimes up to several months in the case of heroin users.

Working with this this client group can provide exceptional challenges when considering these above factors. There is also no published evidence available to indicate the efficacy of the psychobehavioural treatment modalities for insomnia in this group.

Contraindications for REST programme interventions

A number of conditions require considerations that are inappropriate for using the interventions reported in Chapters Five, Six, and Seven of this book, or at least require further investigation before embarking on a programme of psychobehavioural intervention. First, those transient or acute insomnias that might naturally remit with careful "watchful waiting". Often these include an adjustment insomnia, for example, when adjusting to new parenting or another change in life circumstances that might not be considered to be very serious to the individual in question. At the other end of the spectrum are those who are living with particularly serious mental health conditions such as psychosis (despite some initial positive findings for the use of CBTi in this group (Freeman et al., 2015)), where sleep restriction therapy specifically could be potentially hazardous to this client group. In such cases, or indeed if there is any doubt in the mind of the treating healthcare professional when working with a particularly complex presentation, then onward referral to a specialist in behavioural sleep medicine is essential.

Sleep-disordered breathing (examined using the assessment form presented in Chapter Five of this book), from questions relating to severe snoring, high body mass index, excessive daytime sleepiness, and daytime dysfunction, require onward referral (via the client's physician to their local hospitals' respiratory medicine clinic for overnight oximetry). Conducted as an inpatient for a night or two in order to confirm the presence of sleep disordered breathing and its severity. Prescription of a continuous positive airway pressure (CPAP) device to maintain blood oxygen saturation (and reduce hypercapnia) is then often required. Only then should interventions from the REST programme then be considered if problems with sleep persist, but this should not be started until the client has adapted to the use of their CPAP machine (usually a few months after they have been assessed and begun to use the machine.)

Should a client present with suspected narcolepsy (again examined using the assessment form presented in Chapter Five of this book), from questions relating to falling asleep uncontrollably during the day, excessive daytime sleepiness and chronically disturbed sleep. Then they should be referred (again via their physician) to the neurology department of their local hospital for further examination. Only after this referral has been made and met, and after the client has discussed their condition and its management with their neurologist should interventions with the REST programme be considered. If there is a desire from the client to engage in psychobehavioural interventions for their sleep, then close collaboration with their neurologist and physician is also essential.

In any situation where there is concern of significant and imminent risk to the client themselves (e.g., suicidality), or to someone else whom the client may come into contact with (e.g., serious malicious intent), then there is a responsibility of the treating healthcare professional to contact the relevant authorities. Be that the client's physician, or the local accident and emergency department, or indeed, if there is concern about any criminal activity, then the police. Any other interventions should be postponed until any risk factors are no longer of concern.

Summary

This chapter has examined the potential application of psychobehavioural interventions for insomnia in certain groups of clients in order to highlight specific issues that are experienced by these different client groups and the ways in which such interventions can be adjusted and applied effectively for them.

The list of client groups presented here is by no means exhaustive, but the majority of the most commonly presenting conditions are covered. For those not mentioned in this chapter, the adjustments suggested for these different groups should be considered when applying to those not covered in this chapter. Again, where there is doubt or uncertainty, or if REST interventions are contraindicated, then it is always important to tread carefully and discuss with, or refer to, a more experienced professional wherever possible. With careful application, and when a detailed and sensitive assessment of the client has been made, then there is usually much success that can be gained from using the psychobehavioural techniques described earlier in this book. Indeed, as many authors and researchers suggest, where there is a lack of evidence for the use of these approaches within a certain client group, then they are still worth considering because of the wide range of efficacy of these approaches in so many other populations.

CHAPTER SEVEN

Dreams and dreaming

T he final chapter of this book departs from the science of sleep, insomnia, assessment, and treatment strategies; and concludes with an examination of dreams and dreaming. The historical context and current theories as to the purpose and meaning of dreams and dreaming is made in the following sections, before this chapter and book concludes with the application of "dreamwork" in the therapeutic setting.

Background and beginnings in psychotherapy

The origins of dreamwork in psychotherapy begin with Sigmund Freud at the turn of the last century. His famous text *The Interpretation of Dreams* (Freud, 1900) introduced his theory of the unconscious mind through the interpretation of his own, and other people's dreams. Freud regarded dreams as wish fulfilment, in that their purpose is an attempt by the unconscious mind to resolve some conflict or other, either recent or even a long time in the past. He argued that information that is stored in the unconscious mind can be disturbing and potentially destabilising to the conscious mind and that we have a "preconsciousness", which intervenes and prevents such unconscious information breaking through into the consciousness.

With respect to dreams, he postulated that the preconscious becomes less vigilant in this prevention, allowing the unconscious mind to become manifested. His explanation as to the often bizarre, disjointed, and irrational/illogical nature of some dreams was that the preconscious was still effective in a dream state, just not as effective as it is in wakefulness, and the unconscious distorts and changes its form to circumnavigate the barriers of the preconsciousness. Here is where Freud extends his ideas into the interpretation of dreams, as the images that we see (and remember) in our dreams may not be all that they appear to be, and, if they can be interpreted effectively, then they can provide important insights into the subconscious thought-processes of an individual. He described dreams as "the royal road to the unconscious" (Freud, 1900, p. 45).

Freud had his detractors, and much of the criticism levelled at him centred on his tendency to link dream images to body parts, for example caves were linked to the womb, openings of any kind to the vagina, and protrusions, long/slender objects in the dream to the penis. *The Interpretation of Dreams* was also the first time that Freud mentioned his famous idea of the Oedipal complex (Freud, 1900).

Theoretical work in the area was extended by a number of key individuals including Carl Jung who has written widely on symbolism in dreams and extended the idea that dreams maintain an individual's "psychic balance" (Jung, 1933), and Adler who maintained that dreams serve a problem-solving function (Alder, 1927). These psychological theories of dreaming can be subdivided into two broad categories: (1) that the problem-solving function of dreams are to find solutions to cognitive or intellectual problems; and (2) that dreaming is important for emotional regulation or adjustment. Much more recently Antti Revonsuo has argued that any real life event can be regarded as of emotional concern for an individual, and so presents as a problem for psychological adjustment. An idea that dreaming contributes to emotional or behavioural adjustment, which, in turn, is necessary for a solution to an emotional problem (Breger, 1967; Revonsuo in Pace-Schott, Solms, Blagrove, & Harnad, 2000, p. 87).

There are abundant theories as to the purpose of dreams, including wish fulfilment (as mentioned above by Freud in 1900), expectation fulfilment, the continuity hypothesis, the activation–synthesis hypothesis, the threat simulation theory, as well as memory consolidation theories and the concept of the "forgettery" (mentioned in "memory and schemas" in Chapter One of this book). The following sections will briefly expand on these most popular theories as to the purpose of dreams, before a brief critique of them and the current state-of-knowledge in the area before this Chapter concludes with some ideas about the use of dreams and dreaming in the therapeutic context.

Expectation fulfilment

The extension of Freud's idea that dreaming facilitates the "safe" exploration of subconscious wishes, has been put forward by Hans Eysenk, Joe Griffin, and Ivan Tyrell who postulate a more developed theory as to the purpose of dreams, that they have referred to as the expectation-fulfilment theory. The idea here is that during dreaming the brain deactivates, and de-potentiates, unexpressed emotional arousal from prior waking experiences through metaphorical representation and replay. If an insufficient amount of sleep (and so dreaming) has occurred, then an insufficient amount of deactivation of these unexpressed emotions is made, leading to negative psychological consequences the next day, that which we all experience as tiredness and suboptimal functioning when we have not slept well. They also postulate that this serves as a driving mechanism behind the development and maintenance of a range of mental health conditions including depression and anxiety.

This theory supports the circular nature of the development, maintenance and progression of these mental health conditions, as increased emotional arousal during the day (e.g., heightened depressive or anxious mood states) increases the requirement for emotional release during REM sleep, thus depriving the dreamer of the necessary and important slow wave sleep, thus compounding psychological problems for the individual the next day (Griffin & Tyrell, 2014). Possibly by dominant emotional responses (too much REM sleep) and reduced memory consolidation ability (diminished slow wave sleep), from Chapter One.

The continuity hypothesis

The continuity hypothesis of dreaming simply states that dreams are continuous with the waking experiences of the dreamer, and that their waking lives then inspire, inform, and guide their subsequent dreaming.

The idea was first proposed by Calvin Hall in the 1950s (Hall, 1953) and extended more recently by G. William Domhoff in his detailed content analysis of a number of dreams experienced by his subject "Barb Saunders", whose dreams included familiar characters whom she either responded to in a friendly or angry and aggressive way. Her dream manifestations were concordant with her waking interactions as they changed over time with these key people in her life (Domhoff, 2003).

The activation–synthesis hypothesis

First proposed by J. Allan Hobson in 1977 the activation–synthesis hypothesis is a complex neurobiological model of the proposed purpose of dreaming. Much work has been conducted by Hobson and others since the late seventies and an updated model has been put forward—the AIM model, standing for Activation—Input/output gating—Modulation (Hobson, 2010).

The activation element of this model states that in non-REM sleep the brain is largely inactive (with the exception of the hippocampus (for memory consolidation from Chapter One)), but that during wakefulness and in REM sleep the brain becomes reactivated. The input-output gating element states that, despite this reactivation during REM sleep, many functions remain suppressed (e.g., moving—REM sleep-associated paralysis, again from Chapter One) that is, that external sensory input and internal sensory-motor outputs are inhibited. The modulation element has yet to be successfully tested experimentally, but has theoretical merit, in that aminergic and cholinergic neurotransmitters, which are important in the initiation of REM sleep and non-REM sleep, have a widespread influence on many brain regions; and so may be fundamental in the encoding and disintegration of memories, linking with the memory consolidation and "forgettery" theories of the purpose of sleep (from Chapter One again).

Hobson describes brain activation in REM sleep resulting in the synthesis of a dream, and that these are phenomenologically different from the waking experience in that:

1. Dreams are difficult to remember, whereas waking experiences are much easier to remember.
2. Dream content is often quite illogical, more so than waking experiences.

3. There is an "uncritical acceptance" of the dreaming experience, despite their often bizarre content.
4. There are sensory experiences in the dream (without any external input from the environment).
5. Dreams are often associated with extremes of emotion, in excess of the emotional experiences of waking life.

These five phenomena described by Hobson have been supported with experimental data that fit with his AIM model. In that, sensation and emotion in the dream are "activated" by changes in neurotransmission in the brain during sleep, particularly in the limbic regions; and that the suppression of external stimuli, or any motor responses to these internalised dream stimuli, allows stimulation of what he refers to as our "protoconsciousness". An idea that dreaming provides us with an experimental consciousness on which to test, plan, prepare, overlay, rehearse etc. and so to adapt our brains during sleep for more effective functioning whilst we are awake. So, although dreaming is associated with brain activity that is similar to our brains waking activity, it remains phenomenologically different.

The dreaming brain-state may be fundamental for the effective function of this so-called protoconsciousness and that, in order to live functional lives, we need sufficient dreaming to occur to enable our protoconsciousness to set us up for effective conscious activity when we are awake. In other words, although similar in terms of brain activation, dreaming and wakefulness are phenomenologically different, and we need a balanced interaction between the two for the effective function of both (Hobson and colleagues in Pace-Schott, Solms, Blagrove, & Harnad, 2003, p. 50).

Threat simulation theory

Another key player in the debate surrounding the purpose of dreams is Antti Revonsuo who states that the purpose of dreams is to practice the perception and avoidance of environmental threats. If performed optimally, this well-rehearsed, nocturnal practice endows the individual with enhanced threat avoidance skills, which confer an advantage in the ecosystem, and so an increased chance of reproductive success. He reinforces support for this theory, also referred to as an evolutionary theory of dreaming, using empirical evidence from normative dream content, children's dreams (Valli et al., 2005), recurrent dreams, nightmares, post-traumatic dreams, and the dreams of hunter-gatherers, arguing that our dream-production mechanisms are specialised in the simulation of threatening life events (Revonsuo in Pace-Schott, Solms, Blagrove, & Harnad, 2003, p. 85).

Cognitive theory of dreaming

The cognitive theory of dreams was also first proposed by Calvin Hall in the 1950s. Hall stated that dreams were a conceptualisation of our waking experiences. These experiences include perceptions of people in our living environment and ideas of ourselves. This cognitive theory also includes the idea that during dreams we express our creativity (Hall, 1953). He went on to develop the proposition that there are five elements which are present in all of our dreams (Hall & Van de Castle, 1966):

1. Ourselves, including self-regard and our life-roles.
2. Other people and how we act and react towards them.
3. Positive and negative views of the world around us.
4. Morality (i.e., what we consider acceptable and unacceptable as individuals; relating to elements 1, 2, & 3 above).
5. Conflict, both internal and external (again related to elements 1, 2, 3, & 4 above).

As a behaviourist, Hall believed that these conceptual dream elements have a significant impact on how we behave in our waking lives.

David Foulkes has put forward an updated cognitive theory of dreaming. He proposed that dreaming is precipitated by arbitrary and random activation of memory during sleep and that this does not serve any particularly useful adaptive function (Foulkes, 1982). He does, however, make the distinction between the content of dreams and the actual process of dreaming. Although the content may be random and arbitrary, the process itself involves an integration of events (and our sensory experience of them) into what he refers to as a "world ana-logue". In other words, a model of the world that is constructed and actively participated in by the dreamer that incorporates past events (recent or distant). Thus the content of dreams may not be significant, but the process itself may be what is important about them.

In line with Foulkes's assertion that the content of dreams may not have adaptive function Owen Flanagan has, more recently, explicitly refuted the idea that dreams as conscious experiences have any biological function (Flanagan, 1995). His "phenomenal dreaming" (or p-dreaming) hypothesis states that, because no sensory input is processed, or motor output is produced, and that as dreams are arbitrary and random, it is therefore likely that they are an evolutionary remnant. With the only reason that they have survived or persisted within us is that, although they serve no useful purpose, they also do us no harm either.

* * *

This section has examined some of the more popular theories as to the function and purpose of dreaming and identified areas of contention and congruence. There is still much debate as to the true "purpose" of dreaming, or even if dreaming has any purpose at all. The enigmatic nature of dreams makes them very difficult to test in the empirical sense for a number of reasons: First, dreams are very diverse in nature within individuals, let alone between them: at a population level. Second, the recall of dreams is notoriously vague and they are forgotten (usually very quickly) by the dreamer, which makes their capture almost impossible. Third, the measurement of the dream experience has exclusively relied on self-reports, as we do not currently have the technology to capture and record dreams in any objective way. The electrical, magnetic, and chemical impulses that we can measure and analyse tell us next to nothing about what the dreamer is actually experiencing. Fourth, as dreams are internally driven, it is particularly difficult to influence them with external stimulation (see Hobson's input-output gating hypothesis).

So, finally, we are left with a very nebulous understanding of how we can usefully manipulate, control, measure, and interpret dreams in the clinical setting, in such a way as to definitively standardise their use in medicine. However, from a therapeutic perspective, there is little doubt that "dreamwork" can be extremely useful, despite the lack of empirical support for its use, and so the following section will explore the utility of dreams in therapy.

The clinical utility of dreams in therapy

The previous sections of this chapter examined the historical background and the "science" of dreaming, as far as our current understanding permits, putting forward some of the more popular theories on the subject. As we saw, there is still much debate as to the true nature and purpose of the phenomenon of dreaming and, with the lack of any clear definition as to the purpose of dreams, we are at the present time unable to develop testable experimental studies to effectively elucidate the function of dreams, or the process of dreaming. This lack of experimental data leaves us unable to devise evidence-based interventions, which can again be tested for efficacy, and so clinical utility.

As far as having solid evidence-based foundations for "dreamwork" in the therapeutic context is concerned, we are still a long way off. Theory needs to be sound, hypotheses tested, and interventions devised, implemented, and evaluated (with large and diverse groups of people), before we can come close to introducing evidence-based interventions that use dreams and dreaming in the clinical setting. This *a priori*, empiricist approach is what drives our modern health service provision, and so it is very unlikely that referral to a dream-specialist will be available for many years to come, as we are yet to develop any firm consensus on the purpose of dreams even at the theoretical level.

This paints a bleak picture for the use of dreams in therapy, but we do, fortunately, have a lot of anecdotal evidence for their utility and a few empirical studies that have bypassed the lack of theory and have shown some good levels of efficacy in clinical practice (admittedly in only a small number of studies). The second of these refers to the use of imagery rehearsal, already described in previous chapters of this book, which has shown good results in treating children with persistent nightmares and post-traumatic nightmares in veterans (Nappi, Drummond, Thorp, & McQuaid, 2010). The first, the anecdotal evidence, comes from the reports of a large number of therapists whom have been using dreamwork very effectively in their own practices for many decades, going back to the work of Freud over one hundred years ago.

A large number of therapists routinely use dreamwork in their practices, with one survey suggesting that around forty-four per cent of psychoanalysts and fifteen per cent of CBT therapists, regularly using dreamwork (Schredl, Bohusch, Kahl, Mader, & Somesan, 2000). The ability of this book to entertain all the reports of dreamwork by the vast number of practitioners around the world is a challenge beyond these pages, but perhaps best summarised by the work and writings of Irvin D. Yalom.

The chances are that anyone working for any length of time in the world of psychotherapy will have come across Yalom, and if you have not read his work and are in any way involved in therapeutic work, then his books come highly recommended. He writes with erudite compassion and elucidates a very long and successful therapeutic career with modesty and inspirational insight. He has a few things to say about dreams, from his book *The Gift of Therapy: Reflections on Being a Therapist* (Yalom, 2002):

1. Use them, use them, use them.
2. Full interpretation of a dream: forget it!
3. Use dreams pragmatically, pillage and loot.
4. Master some dream navigational skills.
5. Learn about the patient's life from their dreams.
6. Pay attention to the first dream.
7. Attend carefully to dreams about the therapist.

To summarise these ideas of Yalom, one cannot use dreams enough, they can be extremely informative and effective at moving therapy forward especially in breaking through the experience of "getting stuck" with a client in therapy. The totality of a dream is probably not useful, but the elements within them that "speak" can be of particular use, and it is these that need to be tuned into and brought into the therapeutic engagement. Especially feelings, emotions, and key themes (which perhaps map onto Hall's assertions that dreams mirror self-conceptions).

As a therapist, one should take what one needs from the dreams under examination to help with the progression of therapy. With experience the therapist can become more sophisticated, and sensitive, in their use of dreams in therapy, but that this takes time to master. He proposes that much can be learned about the client from their dream experiences and that these insights might often be masked by waking behaviours—again perhaps reflecting Hall's very poignant statement that: "dreams reflect the dreamer's unconscious self-conception, which often does not at all resemble our trumped up and distorted self-portraits by which we fool ourselves in waking life; dreams mirror the self" (Van de Castle, 1994).

There is a school of thought in the therapeutic engagement that initial contacts, first-words spoken, and primary emotional responses, can reflect the core issues that a client may be experiencing (Leiman, 1997). Yalom says that this can also be true for the first dream that a client discloses, as these may be of primary significance to the client and their underlying psychological issues. He also adds a word of warning about being particularly careful about the dreams that the client may have about the therapist, or vice versa, as these may be particularly telling!

A review of dreamwork in psychotherapy conducted by Pesant & Zadra in 2004 identified three types of gains that can be made in the psychotherapeutic engagement by interpreting dreams:

1. Insight (for both the therapist and the client), including seeing one-self in a new light, connecting different aspects of the self, surprise at self-revelation and connexions, and the novelty of the experience.
2. Increased involvement in the process of psychotherapy, including accessing essential or core issues, building a therapeutic relationship, enhanced understanding of client's cognitive style and their behaviour(s) (linked to insight above).
3. Dream content (be that either positive or negative) is essential for interpretation and the progression of therapy, i.e., positive dreams potentially indicate a move towards resolution, and negative dreams can identify problem areas for further focus.

(From: Pesant & Zadra, 2004)

A summary of the theoretical literature on dreaming and the therapeutic utility of dreamwork

The variety and diffuse nature of these numerous theories as to the purpose of dreams indicates the limitations of our current knowledge on the subject as well as the huge number of opportunities that arise for further research. Much has been learned over the last few decades, and, with further technological advances, particularly in the use and application of fMRI it is anticipated that the next decades of research will be a boom-time for dream research. Although there is some contention and there are divergent ideas on the purpose of dreaming, there are also areas of consensus, in summary:

1. Dreams are generated by forebrain mechanisms which can be activated from a number of internal sources, the most common of which is REM sleep arousal, but also limbic and brain stem regions as well (Hobson, Pace-Schott, Stickgold, & Kahn, 1998; Solms 1997).

2. Dreaming is a "cognitive achievement" that develops in childhood (Foulkes, 1999).

3. There is a large amount of support for the memory consolidation and memory disintegration theories of sleep and dreaming, although definitive, empirically tested support for this assertion is still required (Vertes & Eastman in Pace-Schott Solms, Blagrove, & Harnad, 2003, p. 275).

4. Emerging evidence does support, at least at a hypothetical level, the importance of sleep (and therefore dreaming as an integral part of sleep) for memory consolidation and disintegration, the former possibly being related to deep, slow wave non-REM sleep, and the latter to REM sleep, respectively (Landmann et al., 2014).

5. Emotional arousal in dreams is explained by the activation of the limbic regions, especially during REM sleep (Hobson, Pace-Schott, Stickgold, & Kahn, 1998).

6. Although lacking in well-researched, empirical evidence, dreamwork has been reported to be highly effective and widely used in the therapeutic environment (Nappi, Drummond, Thorp, & McQuaid, 2010; Pesant & Zadra, 2004; Yalom, 2002).

This chapter has examined the historical background to the study of dreams and dreaming, put forward some of the more popular historical and contemporaneous theories as to the purpose of dreams and dreaming and briefly described the ways in which dreamwork has been incorporated into the clinical setting. Clearly there is much that remains to be discovered and learned about the elusive and enigmatic phenomenon that are dreams and is the process of dreaming with much promising work in this field inevitable over the coming years, especially with advances in the technology available to us to examine them in more detail.

EPILOGUE

Conclusions

This book began by looking at what sleep is, how it works (to the best of our current understanding), how it changes as we age, and what healthy, normal sleep looks like. We then explored the range of sleeping problems before considering a range of assessment and treatment approaches. The traditional pharmacological and psychobehavioural treatments for insomnia were initially described before a new, second-generation psychobehavioural modality (the REST programme) was introduced. The book then concluded with an examination of how sleep differs for more vulnerable groups, and how the treating healthcare professional might adjust, or attenuate their practice when working with these groups, before the final chapter examined dreams, dreaming, and the utility of dreamwork in therapy.

This book has evolved from a series of workshops and lectures, delivered over the last fifteen years by the author and his colleagues, predominantly to groups of healthcare professionals, but also to interested lay members of the public, some of whom experienced poor sleep. It is to these two groups that this book is essentially aimed, with the hope that the information presented in these pages is not only interesting and informative, but also helpful to improve the sleep of those who read these words; and to those who are dedicated to helping people with whatever conditions that they are trained to manage throughout their careers. The vast number of people who have insomnia in isolation, and as a co-morbidity with other conditions, will therefore have access to this information themselves and also to more experienced clinicians/practitioners who will be well placed to manage their clients' sleep problems as well as their other presenting conditions.

The title of this book: *Teaching the World to Sleep* was amended from the original (less catchy) working title of: "Sleep and insomnia: psychobehavioural assessment and treatment opportunities" for two reasons. First, although the original working title was appropriate and accurate in its description, it was, essentially quite dull. Second, and much more importantly, it is the ambition of the author to spread the word about the contents of this book as widely as possible. It is an intense source of frustration that much of the information presented in this book has been known to the psychological and behavioural sleep sciences for a long time—many of these psychobehavioural techniques have been around for more than thirty years—and yet very few healthcare professionals have received any formalised training in their application, or even awareness of their very existence (beyond simple sleep hygiene) in very many cases. Furthermore, it is disappointing that members of the public, who do not work in the allied health professions, also have very little understanding of sleep and sleep management practices. To the point that millions of people suffer, often quite needlessly, with poor sleep. This has a huge impact, both at an individual level, and at a societal, even global, level; at financial as well as quality of life levels.

We have the technology and we have had it for a long time. The purpose of this book then (and the training courses delivered by the author and his colleagues), is to join this technology to those people who need it (either through their work with clients, or in their own bedrooms at night), to help the world to sleep.

REFERENCES

Adler, A. (1927). *The Practice and Theory of Individual Psychology.* New York, NY: Harcourt Inc.

Ahmed, I., & Thorpy, M. (2010). Clinical features, diagnosis and treatment of narcolepsy. *Clinics in Chest Medicine, 31:* 371–381.

Åkerstedt, T., Kecklund, G., Ingre, M., Lekander, M., & Axelsson, J. (2009). Sleep homeostasis during repeated sleep restriction and recovery: Support from EEG dynamics. *Sleep, 32:* 217–222.

Alberti, A. (2014). Sleep changes. *Frontiers of Neurology and Neuroscience, 30:* 38–40.

Aldabal, L., & Bahammam, A. S. (2011). Metabolic, endocrine, and immune consequences of sleep deprivation. *The Open Respiratory Medicine Journal, 5:* 31–43.

Allen, S. L., Howlett, M. D., Coulombe, J. A., & Corkum, P. V. (2015). ABCs of SLEEPING: A review of the evidence behind pediatric sleep practice recommendations. *Sleep Medicine Reviews, 29:* 1–14.

American Psychiatric Association (2013). *Sleep Wake Disorders. Diagnostic and Statistical Manual of Mental Disorders: DSM-5.* (5th Edition). Washington, DC: American Psychiatric Association.

American Sleep Disorders Association (ASDA) report (1995). Practice parameters for the use of actigraphy in the clinical assessment of sleep disorders. *Sleep, 18:* 285–287.

Arendt, J. (2000). Melatonin, circadian rhythms, and sleep. *New England Journal of Medicine, 343*: 1114–1116.

Asada, T., Motonaga, T., Yamagata, Z., Uno, M., & Takahashi, K. (2000). Associations between retrospectively recalled napping behavior and later development of Alzheimer's disease: association with APOE genotypes. *Sleep, 23*: 629–634.

Aschoff, J., Fatranská, M., Giedke, H., Doerr, P., Stamm, D., & Wisser, H. (1971). Human circadian rhythms in continuous darkness: entrainment by social cues. *Science, 171*: 213–215.

Ashton, C. H. (1997). Benzodiazepine dependency. In: A. Baum, S. Newman, J. Weinman, R. West, & C. McManus (Eds)., *Cambridge Handbook of Psychology & Medicine* (pp. 376–380). Cambridge: Cambridge University Press.

Ashton, C. H. (2002). The Ashton Manual. www.benzo.org/manual/index [Last accessed 9 October 2015].

Auger, R. R. (2006). Sleep-related eating disorders. *Psychiatry, 3*: 64–70.

Aurora, R. N., Kristo, D. A., Bista, S. R., Rowley, J. A., Zak, R. S., Casey, K. R., Lamm, C. I., Tracy, S. L., & Rosenberg, R. S.; American Academy of Sleep Medicine. (2012). The treatment of restless legs syndrome and periodic limb movement disorder in adults—an update for 2012: Practice parameters with an evidence-based systematic review and meta-analyses: an American Academy of Sleep Medicine Clinical Practice Guideline. *Sleep, 35*: 1039–1062.

Bakshi, R., Shaikh, Z. A., Miletich, R. S., Czarnecki, D., Dmochowski, J., & Henschel, K. (2000). Fatigue in multiple sclerosis and its relationship to depression and neurologic disability. *Multiple Sclerosis, 6*: 181–185.

Barbera, J., & Shapiro, C. (2005). Benefit-risk assessment of zaleplon in the treatment of insomnia. *Drug Safety, 28*: 301–318.

Baron, K. G., Corden, M., Jin, L., & Mohr, D. C. (2011). Impact of psychotherapy on insomnia symptoms in patients with depression and multiple sclerosis. *Journal of Behavioral Medicine, 34*: 92–101.

Bassetti, C. L. (2005). Sleep and stroke. *Seminars in Neurology, 25*(1): 19–32.

Bastien, C. H., Turcotte, I., St-Jean, G., Morin, C. M., & Carrier, J. (2013). Information processing varies between insomnia types: measures of N1 and P2 during the night. *Behavioral Sleep Medicine, 11*(1): 56–72.

Belleville, G., Cousineau, H., Levrier, K., & St-Pierre-Delorme, M. È. (2011). Meta-analytic review of the impact of cognitive-behavior therapy for insomnia on concomitant anxiety. *Clinical Psychology Reviews, 31*: 638–652.

Bes, F., Schulz, H., Navelet, Y., & Salzarulo, P. (1991). The distribution of slow-wave sleep across the night: a comparison for infants, children, and adults. *Sleep, 14*(1): 5–12.

Bested, A. C., & Marshall, L. M. (2015). Review of Myalgic Encephalomyelitis/ Chronic Fatigue Syndrome: an evidence-based approach to diagnosis and management by clinicians. *Reviews on Environmental Health, 30*: 223–249.

Bixler, E. O., Papaliaga, M. N., Vgontzas, A. N., Lin, H. M., Pejovic, A., Karataraki, M., Vela-Bueno, A., & Chrousos, G. P. (2009). Women sleep objectively better than men and the sleep of young women is more resilient to external stressors: effects of age and menopause. *Journal of Sleep Research, 18*: 221–228.

Bliwise, D. L. (1993). Sleep in normal ageing and dementia—a review. *Sleep, 16*(1): 40–81.

Blood, M., Sack, R., Percy, D., & Pen, J. (1997). A comparison of sleep detection by wrist actigraphy, behavioural response and polysomnography. *Sleep, 20*: 388–395.

Boeve, B. F., Silber, M. H., & Ferman, T. J. (2004). REM sleep behavior disorder in Parkinson's disease and dementia with Lewy bodies. *Journal of Geriatric Psychiatry and Neurology, 17*: 146–157.

Bootzin, R. R. (1972). Stimulus control treatment for insomnia. *Proceedings of the American Psychological Association, 7*: 395–396.

Bradbury, S., Principal Deputy Assistant Attorney General, Office of Legal Counsel (2005). Re: Application of 18 U.S.C. 2340-2340A to certain techniques that may be used in the interrogation of a high value al Qaeda detainee. Memorandum for John A. Rizzo, Senior Deputy General Counsel, Central Intelligence Agency, 10 May 2005.

Bradley, T. D., & Phillipson, E. A. (1992). Central sleep apnea. *Clinics in Chest Medicine 13*: 493–505.

Breger, L. (1967). Function of dreams. *Journal of Abnormal Psychology Monograph, 72*: 1–28.

Brooks, A. T., & Wallen, G. R. (2014). Sleep disturbances in individuals with alcohol-related disorders: A review of cognitive-behavioral therapy for insomnia (CBT-I) and associated non-pharmacological therapies. *Substance Abuse, 16*: 55–62.

Bruni, O., & Novelli, L. (2010). Sleep disorders in children. *British Medical Journal Clinical Evidence, pii*: 2304.

Bruni. O., Alonso-Alconada, D., Besag, F., Biran, V., Braam, W., Cortese, S., Moavero, R., Parisi, P., Smits, M., Van der Heijden, K., & Curatolo, P. (2015). Current role of melatonin in pediatric neurology: clinical recommendations. *European Journal of Paediatric Neurology, 19*: 122–133.

Buysee, D., Reynolds, C., Monk, T., Berman, S., & Kupfer, D. (1989). The pittsburgh sleep quality index: A new instrument for psychiatric practice and research. *Psychiatry Research, 28*: 193–213.

Buzzi, G., & Cirignotta, F. (2000). Isolated sleep paralysis: a web survey. *Sleep Research Online, 3*: 61–66.

Carskadon, M. A., & Dement, W. C. (1982). The multiple sleep latency test: what does it measure? *Sleep, 5*: S67–S72.

Chambers, M., & Alexander, S. (1992). Assessment and prediction of outcome for a brief behavioural insomnia treatment program. *Journal of Behavioural Therapeutic Experimental Psychiatry, 23*: 289–297.

Chang, J. J., Pien, G. W., Duntley, S. P., & Macones, G. A. (2010). Sleep deprivation during pregnancy and maternal and fetal outcomes: is there a relationship? *Sleep Medicine Reviews, 14*: 107–114.

Cheng, S. K., & Dizon, J. (2012). Computerised cognitive behavioural therapy for insomnia: a systematic review and meta-analysis. *Psychotherapy and Psychosomatics, 81*: 206–216.

Chester, G. B. (1985). Influence of analgesic drugs in road crashes. *Annals of Accident Prevention, 135*: 303–309.

Clancy, M., Drerup, M., & Sullivan, A. B. (2015). Outcomes of cognitive-behavioral treatment for insomnia on insomnia, depression, and fatigue for individuals with multiple sclerosis: A case series. *International Journal of Multiple Sclerosis Care, 17*: 261– 267.

Cole, R., Kripke, D., Gruen, W., Mullaney, D., & Gillin, J. (1992). Automatic sleep/wake identification from wrist activity. *Sleep, 15*: 461–491.

Costa, G. (1996). The impact of shift and night work on health. *Applied Ergonomics, 27*(1): 9–16.

Czeisler, C. A., Duffy, J. F., Shanahan, T. L., Brown, E. N., Mitchell, J. F., Rimmer, D. W., Ronda, J. M., Silva, E. J., Allan, J. S., Emens, J. S., Dijk, D. J., & Kronauer, R. E. (1999). Stability, precision, and near-24-hour period of the human circadian pacemaker. *Science, 284*: 2177– 2181.

Czeisler, C. A., Zimmerman, J. C., Ronda, J. M., Moore-Ede, M. C., & Weitzman, E. D. (1980). Timing of REM sleep is coupled to the circadian rhythm of body temperature in man. *Sleep, 2*: 329–346.

Dauvilliers, Y., Arnulf, I., & Mignot, E. (2007). Narcolepsy with cataplexy. *Lancet, 369*: 499–511.

David, R., Zeitzer, J., Friedman, L., Noda, A., O'Hara, R., Robert, P., & Yesavage, J. A. (2010). Non-pharmacologic management of sleep disturbance in Alzheimer's disease. *Journal of Nutrition Health and Aging, 14*: 203–206.

Davis, S., Mirick, D. K., & Stevens, R. G. (2001). Night shift work, light at night and risk of breast cancer. *Journal of the National Cancer Institute, 93*: 1557–1562.

de Jonghe, A., Korevaar, J. C., van Munster, B. C., & de Rooij, S. E. (2010). Effectiveness of melatonin treatment on circadian rhythm disturbances in dementia. Are there implications for delirium? A systematic review. *International Journal of Geriatric Psychiatry, 25*: 1201–1208.

DiBianco, J. M., Morley, C., & Al-Omar, O. (2014). Nocturnal enuresis: A topic review and institution experience. *Avicenna Journal of Medicine*, 4: 77–86.

Dijk, D. J., Duffy, J. F., & Czeisler, C. A. (2000). Contribution of circadian physiology and sleep homeostasis to age-related changes in human sleep. *Chronobiology International*, 17: 285–311.

Dodson, E. R., & Zee, P. C. (2010). Therapeutics for circadian rhythm sleep disorders. *Sleep Medicine Clinics*, 5: 701–715.

Domhoff, G. W. (2003). *The Scientific Study of Dreams: Neural Networks, Cognitive Development, and Content Analysis*. Washington, DC: American Psychological Association.

Donga, E., van Dijk, M., van Dijk, J. G., Biermasz, N. R., Lammers, G. J., van Kralingen, K. W., Corssmit, E. P., & Romijn, J. A. (2010). A single night of partial sleep deprivation induces insulin resistance in multiple metabolic pathways in healthy subjects. *Journal of Clinical Endocrinology and Metabolism*, 95: 2963–2968.

Espie, C. A. (2006). *Overcoming Insomnia and Sleep Problems. A Self-Help Guide Using Cognitive Behavioral Techniques*. London: Constable and Robinson.

Espie, C. A. (2009). "Stepped care": a health technology solution for delivering cognitive behavioral therapy as a first line insomnia treatment. *Sleep*, 32: 1549–1558.

Espie, C. A., Broomfield, N. M., MacMahon, K. M., Macphee, L. M., & Taylor, L. M. (2006). The attention-intention-effort pathway in the development of psychophysiologic insomnia: a theoretical review. *Sleep Medicine Reviews*, 10: 215–245.

Espie, C. A., Inglis, S. J., Tessuer, S., & Harvey, L. (2001). The clinical effectiveness of cognitive behaviour therapy for chronic insomnia: implementation and evaluation of a sleep clinic in general medical practice. *Behaviour Research and Therapy*, 39(1): 45–60.

Espie, C. A., Kyle, S. D., Williams, C., Ong, J. C., Douglas, N. J., Hames, P., & Brown, J. S. L. (2012). A randomized, placebo-controlled trial of online cognitive behavioral therapy for chronic insomnia disorder delivered via an automated media-rich web application. *Sleep*, 35: 769–781.

Espie, C. A., MacMahon, K. M., Kelly, H. L., Broomfield, N. M., Douglas, N. J., Engleman, H. M., McKinstry, B., Morin, C. M., Walker, A., & Wilson, P. (2007). Randomized clinical effectiveness trial of nurse-administered small-group cognitive behavior therapy for persistent insomnia in general practice. *Sleep*, 30: 574–584.

Evans, B. M., & Bartlett, J. R. (1995). Prediction of outcome in severe head injury based on recognition of sleep related activity in the polygraphic electroencephalogram. *Journal of Neurology, Neurosurgery and Psychiatry*, 59(1): 17–25.

Ferber, R. (2013). *Solve your Child's Sleep Problems.* 2nd Edition. London: Vermillion.

Fernandez-Mendoza, J., Calhoun, S. L., Bixler, E. O., Karataraki, M., Liao, D., Vela-Bueno, A., Jose Ramos-Platon, M., Sauder, K. A., Basta, M., & Vgontzas, A. N. (2011). Sleep misperception and chronic insomnia in the general population: role of objective sleep duration and psychological profiles. *Psychosomatic Medicine, 73*(1): 88–97.

Finan, P. H., Buenaver, L. F., Coryell, V. T., & Smith, M. T. (2014). Cognitive-behavioral therapy for comorbid insomnia and chronic pain. *Sleep Medicine Clinics, 9*: 261–274.

Finkbeiner, A. (2014). Awake asleep: Insomniac brains that can't switch off. *New Scientist, 2969*: 34.

Flanagan, O. (1995). Deconstructing dreams: The spandrels of sleep. *The Journal of Philosophy, 92*(1): 5–27.

Foulkes, D. (1982). A cognitive-psychological model of REM dream production. *Sleep, 5*: 169–187.

Foulkes, D. (1999). *Children's Dreaming and the Development of Consciousness.* Cambridge, MA: Harvard University Press.

Frankl, V. (1959). *Man's Search for Meaning* (1984 ed.). New York, NY: Simon & Schuster.

Freeman, D., Waite, F., Startup, H., Myers, E., Lister, R., McInerney, J, Harvey, A. G., Geddes, J., Zaiwalla, Z., Luengo-Fernandez, R., Foster, R., Clifton, L., & Yu, L. M. (2015). Efficacy of cognitive behavioural therapy for sleep improvement in patients with persistent delusions and hallucinations (BEST): a prospective, assessor-blind, randomised controlled pilot trial. *Lancet Psychiatry, 2*: 975–983.

Frese, A., Summ, O., & Evers, S. (2014). Exploding head syndrome: six new cases and review of the literature. *Cephalalgia, 34*: 823–827.

Freud, S. (1900). *The Interpretation of Dreams.* (J. Strachey, Trans. Ed. (1955)). New York: Basic Books.

Friedman, L., Bliwise, D., Yesavage, J., & Salom, S. (1991). A preliminary study comparing sleep restriction and relaxation treatments for insomnia in older adults. *Journal of Gerontology, 46*: 1–8.

Garcia-Rill, E., Luster, B., Mahaffey, S., Bisagno, V., & Urbano, F. J. (2015). Pedunculopontine arousal system physiology—Implications for insomnia. *Sleep Science, 8*: 92–99.

Gibson, G. J. (2007). Obstructive sleep apnoea syndrome: underestimated and undertreated. *British Medical Bulletin, 72*: 49–65.

Gominak, S. C., & Stumpf, W. E. (2012). The world epidemic of sleep disorders is linked to vitamin D deficiency. *Medical Hypotheses, 79*: 132–135.

Griffin, J., & Tyrell, I. (2014). *Why we Dream: The Definitive Answer.* Chalvington, East Sussex: HG Publishing.

Gringras, P., Middleton, B., Skene, D. J., & Revell, V. L. (2015). Bigger, Brighter, Bluer-Better? Current Light-Emitting Devices—Adverse Sleep Properties and Preventative Strategies. *Frontiers in Public Health*, 3: 233.

Guarnieri, B., & Sorbi, S. (2015). Sleep and Cognitive Decline: A Strong Bidirectional Relationship. It is time for specific recommendations on routine assessment and the management of sleep disorders in patients with mild cognitive impairment and dementia. *European Neurology*, 74: 43–48.

Guénolé, F., Godbout, R., Nicolas, A., Franco, P., Claustrat, B., & Baleyte, J. M. (2011). Melatonin for disordered sleep in individuals with autism spectrum disorders: systematic review and discussion. *Sleep Medicine Reviews 15*: 379–387.

Guilleminault, C., Hagen, C. C., & Khaja, A. M. (2008). Catathrenia: parasomnia or uncommon feature of sleep disordered breathing? *Sleep, 31*(1): 132–139.

Gulevich, G., Dement, W., & Johnson, L. (1966). Psychiatric and EEG observations on a case of prolonged (264 hours) wakefulness. *Archives of General Psychiatry, 15*(1): 29–35.

Hall, C. S. (1953). A cognitive theory of dreams. *Journal of General Psychology, 49*: 273–282.

Hall, C. S., & Van de Castle, R. I. (1966). *The Content Analysis of Dreams*. New York, NY: Appleton-Century-Crofts.

Harvey, A. G. (2002). A cognitive model of insomnia. *Behavioural Research and Therapy, 40*: 869–893.

Haupt, M., Sheldon, S. H., & Loghmanee, D. (2013). Just a scary dream? A brief review of sleep terrors, nightmares, and rapid eye movement sleep behavior disorder. *Pediatric Annals, 42*: 211–216.

Hauri, P. J. (1998). Insomnia. *Clinics in Chest Medicine, 19*(1): 157–159.

Hauri, P. J., Hayes, B., Sateia, M., Hellekson, C., Percy, L., & Olmstead, E. (1982). Effectiveness of a sleep disorders centre—a 9-month follow-up. *American Journal of Psychiatry, 139*: 663–666.

Hedman, C., Pohjasvaara, T., Tolonen, U., Suhonen-Malm, A. S., & Myllylä, V. V. (2002). Effects of pregnancy on mothers' sleep. *Sleep Medicine, 3*(1): 37–42.

Hertz, G., Fast, A., Feinsilver, S. H., Albertario, C. L., Schulman, H., & Fein, A. M. (1992). Sleep in normal late pregnancy. *Sleep, 15*: 246–251.

Hobson, J. A. (2010). REM sleep and dreaming: Towards a theory of proto-consciousness. *Nature Reviews Neuroscience, 10*: 803–813.

Hobson, J. A., Pace-Schott, E. F., Stickgold, R., & Kahn, D. (1998). To dream or not to dream? Relevant data from new neuroimaging and electrophysiological studies. *Current Opinion in Neurobiology, 8*: 239–244.

Horne, J. A., & Ostberg, O. (1976). A self-assessment questionnaire to determine morningness-eveningness in human circadian rhythms. *International Journal of Chronobiology, 4*: 97–110.

Huang, W., Shah, S., Long, Q., Crankshaw, A. K., & Tanphysicianricha, V. (2013). Improvement of pain, sleep, and quality of life in chronic pain patients with vitamin D supplementation. *Clinical Journal of Pain, 29*: 341–347.

Iber, C., Ancoli-Israel, S., Chesson, A., & Quan, S. F., for the American Academy of Sleep Medicine (2007). *The AASM Manual for the Scoring of Sleep and Associated Events: Rules, Terminology and Technical Specifications.* Westchester: American Academy of Sleep Medicine.

Irish, L. A., Kline, C. E., Gunn, H. E., Buysse, D. J. & Hall, M. H. (2014). The role of sleep hygiene in promoting public health: A review of empirical evidence. *Sleep Medicine Reviews, 22*: 23–36.

Jacobs, G. D., Pace-Schott, E. F., Stickgold, R., & Otto, M. W. (2004). Cognitive behavior therapy and pharmacotherapy for insomnia: a randomized controlled trial and direct comparison. *Archives of Internal Medicine, 164*: 1888–1896.

Jain, F. A., Nazarian, N., & Lavretsky, H. (2014). Feasibility of central meditation and imagery therapy for dementia caregivers. *International Journal of Geriatric Psychiatry, 29*: 870–876.

Joffe, H., Massler, A., & Sharkey, K. M. (2010). Evaluation and management of sleep disturbance during the menopause transition. *Seminars in Reproductive Medicine, 28*: 404–421.

Johns, M. W. (1991). A new method for measuring daytime sleepiness—the Epworth Sleepiness Scale. *Sleep, 14*: 540–545.

Jung, C. G. (1933). *Modern Man in Search of a Soul.* New York, NY: Harcourt Inc.

Kesselring, A., Krulik, T., Bichsel, M., Minder, C., Beck, J. C., & Stuck, A. E. (2001). Emotional and physical demands on caregivers in home care to the elderly in Switzerland and their relationship to nursing home admission. *European Journal of Public Health, 11*: 267–273.

Klein, D., Steinberg, M., Galik, E., Steele, C., Sheppard, J., Warren, A., Rosenblatt, A., & Lyketsos, C. (1999). Wandering behaviour in community residing persons with dementia. *International Journal of Geriatric Psychiatry, 14*: 272–279.

Krakowiak, P., Goodlin-Jones, B., Hertz-Picciotto, I., Croen, L. A., & Hansen, R. L. (2008). Sleep problems in children with autism spectrum disorders, developmental delays, and typical development: a population-based study. *Journal of Sleep Research, 17*: 197–206.

Lac, G., & Chamoux, A. (2004). Biological and psychological responses to two rapid shiftwork schedules. *Ergonomics, 47*: 1339–1349.

Lacks, P., & Morin, C. M. (1992). Recent advances in the assessment and treatment of insomnia. *Journal of Consulting and Clinical Psychology, 60*: 586–594.

Lader, M. (2011). Benzodiazepines revisited—will we ever learn? *Addiction, 106*: 2086–2109.

Lader, M., Tylee, A., & Donoghue, J. (2009). Withdrawing benzodiazepines in primary care. *CNS Drugs, 23*(1): 19–34.

Ladouceur, R., & Gros-Louis, Y. (1986). Paradoxical intention vs stimulus control in the treatment of severe insomnia. *Journal of Behaviour Therapy and Experimental Psychiatry, 17*: 267–269.

Landmann, N., Kuhn, M., Piosczyk, H., Feige, B., Baglioni, C., Spiegelhalder, K., Frase, L., Riemann, D., Sterr, A., & Nissen, C. (2014). The reorganisation of memory during sleep. *Sleep Medicine Reviews, 18*: 531–541.

Lands, W. E. (1999). Alcohol, slow wave sleep, and the somatotropic axis. *Alcohol, 18*: 109–122.

Lee, D. R. (2015). Chapter six: Managing sleep in pregnancy. In: J. Wilks, *Choices in Pregnancy and Childbirth* (pp. 77–82). London and Philadelphia: Singing Dragon Publishing.

Lee, D. R., Morgan, K., & Lindesay, J. E. B. (2004). Impact of respite care on sleep disturbance in dementia caregiving. *Journal of Sleep Research, 13*: 515.

Lee, D. R., Morgan, K., & Lindesay, J. E. B. (2007). The impact of respite care on the sleep of older people with dementia and their caregivers. *Journal of the American Geriatrics Society, 55*: 252–258.

Lee, D. R., Newell, R., Ziegler, L., & Topping, A. (2008). Treatment of fatigue in multiple sclerosis: a systematic review of the literature. *International Journal of Nursing Practice, 14*: 81–93.

Leiman, M. (1997). Procedures as dialogical sequences: a revised version of the fundamental concept in cognitive analytic therapy. *British Journal of Medical Psychology, 70*: 193–207.

Leschziner, G., & Gringras, P. (2012). Restless legs syndrome. *British Medical Journal, 344*: e3056.

Lindemann, R., & Bondemark, L. (2001). A review of oral devices in the treatment of habitual snoring and obstructive sleep apnoea. *Swedish Dental Journal, 25*(1): 39–51.

Little, S. E., McNamara, C. J., & Miller, R. C. (2014). Sleep changes in normal pregnancy. *Obstetric Gynaecology, 123*(1): 153S.

Livingston, G., Manela, M., & Katona, C. (1996). Depression and other psychiatric morbidity in carers of elderly people living at home. *British Medical Journal, 312*: 153–156.

Maguire, E. A., Gadian, D. G., Johnsrude, I. S., Good, C. D., Ashburner, J., Frackowiak, R. S., & Frith, C. D. (2000). Navigation-related structural change in the hippocampi of taxi drivers. *Proceeds of the National Academy of Sciences of the United States of America, 97*: 4398–4403.

Manber, R., Edinger, J. D., Gress, J. L., San Pedro-Salcedo, M. G., Kuo, T. F., & Kalista, T. (2008). Cognitive behavioral therapy for insomnia enhances depression outcome in patients with comorbid major depressive disorder and insomnia. *Sleep, 31*: 489–495.

Massa, J., Stone, K. L., Wei, E. K., Harrison, S. L., Barrett-Connor, E., Lane, N. E., Paudel, M., Redline, S., Ancoli-Israel, S., Orwoll, E., & Schernhammer, E. (2015). Vitamin D and actigraphic sleep outcomes in older community-dwelling men: the MrOS Sleep Study. *Sleep, 38*: 251–257.

McDonald, J. P. (2003). A review of surgical treatment for obstructive sleep apnoea/hypopnoea syndrome. *Surgeon, 5*: 259–264.

Michelini, S., Cassano, G. B., Frare, F., & Perugi, G. (1996). Long-term use of benzodiazepines: tolerance, dependence and clinical problems in anxiety and mood disorders. *Pharmacopsychiatry, 29*: 127–134.

Mindell, J. A., & Jacobson, B. J. (2000). Sleep disturbances during pregnancy. *Journal of Obstetric Gynaecology and Neonatal Nursing, 29*: 590–597.

Minges, K. E., & Redeker, N. S. (2016). Delayed school start times and adolescent sleep: A systematic review of the experimental evidence. *Sleep Medicine Reviews, 28*: 82–91.

Mitchell, M. D., Gehrman, P., Perlis, M., & Umscheid, C. A. (2012). Comparative effectiveness of cognitive behavioral therapy for insomnia: a systematic review. *BMC Family Practice, 25*: 13–40.

Mitchell, U. H. (2011). Nondrug-related aspect of treating Ekbom disease, formerly known as restless legs syndrome. *Neuropsychiatric Disease and Treatment, 7*: 251–257.

Montgomery, P., & Denis, J. (2004). A systematic review of non-pharmacological therapies for sleep problems in later life. *Sleep Medicine Reviews, 8*(1): 47–62.

Moore-Ede, M. C., Sulzman, F. M., & Fuller, C. A. (1982). *The Clocks That Time Us*. Cambridge, Massachusetts, MA: Harvard University Press.

Morgenthaler, T., Kramer, M., Alessi, C., Friedman, L., Boehlecke, B., Brown, T., Coleman, J., Kapur, V., Lee-Chiong, T., Owens, J., Pancer, J., & Swick, T. (2006). Practice parameters for the psychological and behavioral treatment of insomnia: an update. An American Academy of Sleep Medicine report. *Sleep, 29*: 1415–1419.

Morin, C. M. (2003). *Insomnia: A Clinician's Guide to Assessment and Treatment*. New York, NY: Kluwer Academic/Plenum Publishers.

Morin, C. M., Bootzin, R. R., Buysse, D. J., Edinger, J. D., Espie, C. A., & Lichstein, K. L. (2006). Psychological and behavioral treatment of insomnia: Update of the recent evidence (1998–2004) (AASM taskforce review). *Sleep, 29*: 1398–1414.

Morin, C. M., Hauri, P. J., Espie, C. A., Spielman, A. J., Buysse, D. J., & Bootzin, R. R. (1999). Nonpharmacologic treatment of chronic insomnia. *Sleep, 22*: 1134–1157.

Morin, C.M., Kowatch, R., & O'Shanick, G. (1990). Sleep restriction for the inpatient treatment of insomnia. *Sleep* 13(2): 183–186.

Morrison, I., Rumbold, J. M., & Riha, R. L. (2014). Medicolegal aspects of complex behaviours arising from the sleep period: a review and guide for the practising sleep physician. *Sleep Medicine Reviews, 18*: 249–260.

Murali, R. V., Rangarajan, P., & Mounissamy, A. (2015). Bruxism: Conceptual discussion and review. *Journal of Pharmacy and Bioallied Sciences,* 1: S265–S270.

Nappi, C. M., Drummond, S. P., Thorp, S. R., & McQuaid, J. R. (2010). Effectiveness of imagery rehearsal therapy for the treatment of combat-related nightmares in veterans. *Behavior Therapy, 41*: 237–244.

National Institute for Health and Care Excellence. (2016). Clinical Knowledge Summaries. http://cks.nice.org.uk/insomnia#!scenariorecommendation:2 [last accessed 17 June 2016].

Nedeltcheva, A. V., & Scheer, F. A. (2014). Metabolic effects of sleep disruption, links to obesity and diabetes. *Current Opinion in Endocrinology Diabetes and Obesity, 21*: 293–298.

Okawa, M., & Uchiyama, M. (2007). Circadian rhythm sleep disorders: characteristics and entrainment pathology in delayed sleep phase and non-24 sleep–wake syndrome. *Sleep Medicine Reviews, 11*: 485–496.

Ouellet, M. C., Beaulieu-Bonneau, S., & Morin, C. M. (2015). Sleep-wake disturbances after traumatic brain injury. *Lancet Neurology, 14*: 746–757.

Ouellet, M. C., & Morin, C. M. (2004). Cognitive behavioral therapy for insomnia associated with traumatic brain injury: a single-case study. *Archives of. Physical Medicine and Rehabilitation, 85*: 1298–1302.

Pace-Schott, E. F., Solms, M., Blagrove, M., & Harnad, S. (Eds.) (2003). *Sleep and Dreaming Scientific Advances and Reconsiderations.* Cambridge: Cambridge University Press.

Pearce, J. M. (1989). Clinical features of the exploding head syndrome. *Journal of Neurology Neurosurgery and Psychiatry, 52*: 907–910.

Perlis, M. L., Jungquist, C., Smith, M. T., & Posner, D. (2008). *Insomnia: A Session by Session Guide.* 2nd edition. New York, NY: Springer.

Pesant, N., & Zadra, A. (2004). Working with dreams in therapy: what do we know and what should we do? *Clinical Psychology Reviews, 24*: 489–512.

Phillips, B., Cook, Y., Schmitt, F., & Berry, D. (1989). Sleep apnea: prevalence of risk factors in a general population. *Southern Medical Journal, 82*: 1090–1092.

Pigeon, W. R., Moynihan, J., Matteson-Rusby, S., Jungquist, C. R., Xia, Y., Tu, X., & Perlis, M. L. (2012). Comparative Effectiveness of CBT Interventions for Co-Morbid Chronic Pain & Insomnia: A Pilot Study. *Behaviour Research and Therapy, 50*: 685–689.

Pires, G. N., Andersen, M. L., Giovenardi, M., & Tufik, S. (2010). Sleep impairment during pregnancy: possible implications on mother–infant relationship. *Medical Hypotheses, 75*: 578–582.

Prigatano, G. P., Stahl, M. L., Orr, W. C., & Zeiner, H. K. (1982). Sleep and dreaming disturbances in closed head injury patients. *Journal of Neurology, Neurosurgery and Psychiatry, 45*(1): 78–80.

Putilov, A., Donskaya, O., & Verevkin, E. (2015). How many diurnal types are there? A search for two further "bird species". *Personality and Individual Differences, 72:* 12–17.

Rajaratnam, S. M., & Arendt, J. (2001). Health in a 24-h society. *Lancet, 358:* 999–1005.

Rechtschaffen, A., & Kales, A. (1968). *A Manual of Standardised Terminology, Techniques and Scoring System of Sleep Stages in Human Subjects,* Los Angeles: UCLA Brain Information Service.

Riemann, D., Kloepfer, C., & Berger, M. (2009). Functional and structural brain alterations in insomnia: implications for pathophysiology. *European Journal of Neuroscience, 29:* 1754–1760.

Riemann, D., Spiegelhalder, K., Feige, B., Vodeholzer, U., Berger, M., & Perils, M. (2010). The hyperarousal model of insomnia: a review of the concept and its evidence. *Sleep Medicine Reviews, 14:* 19–31.

Ritterband, L. M., Thorndike, F. P., Gonder-Frederick, L. A., Magee, J. C., Bailey, E., Saylor, D. K., & Morin, C. M. (2009). Efficacy of an internet-based behavioral intervention for adults with insomnia. *Archives of General Psychiatry, 66:* 692–698.

Roffwarg, H. P., Muzio, J. N., & Dement, W. C. (1966). Ontogenetic development of the human sleep-dream cycle. *Science, 152:* 604–619.

Roth, T., Coulouvrat, C., Hajak, G., Lakoma, M. D., Sampson, N. A., Shahly, V., Shillington, A. C., Stephenson, J. J., Walsh, J. K., & Kessler, R. C. (2011). Prevalence and perceived health associated with insomnia based on DSM-IV-TR; international statistical classification of diseases and related health problems, tenth revision; and research diagnostic criteria/international classification of sleep disorders, second edition criteria: results from the america insomnia survey. *Biological Psychiatry, 69:* 592–600.

Ruttan, L., Martin, K., Liu, A., Colella, B., & Green, R. E. (2008). Long-term cognitive outcome in moderate to severe traumatic brain injury: a meta-analysis examining timed and untimed tests at 1 and 4.5 or more years after injury. *Archives of Physical Medicine and Rehabilitation, 89:* S69–S76.

Sack, R. L., Auckley, D., Auger, R. R., Carskadon, M. A., Wright, K. P. Jr., Vitiello, M. V., & Zhdanova, I. V. (2007). Circadian rhythm sleep disorders: part II, advanced sleep phase disorder, delayed sleep phase disorder, free-running disorder, and irregular sleep–wake rhythm. An american academy of sleep medicine review. *Sleep, 30:* 1484–1501.

Sadeh, A. (2005). Cognitive-behavioral treatment for childhood sleep disorders. *Clinical Psychology Review, 25:* 612–628.

Sánchez-Ortuño, M. M., & Edinger, J. D. (2012). Cognitive-behavioral therapy for the management of insomnia comorbid with mental disorders. *Current Psychiatry Reports, 14*: 519–528.

Schenck, C. H. (2005). *Paradox Lost—Midnight In The Battleground Of Sleep And Dreams—Violent Moving Nightmares, REM Sleep Behavior Disorder.* Janesville, WI: Extreme-Nights LLC. ISBN-13: 9780976373407.

Schenck, C. H., & Mahowald, M. W. (1994). Review of nocturnal sleep-related eating disorders. *International Journal of Eating Disorders, 15*: 343–356.

Schernhammer, E. S., Laden, F., Speizer, F. E., Willett, W. C., Hunter, D. J., Kawachi, I., Fuchs, C. S., & Colditz, G. A. (2003). Night-shift work and risk of colorectal cancer in the nurses' health study. *Journal of the National Cancer Institute, 95*: 825–828.

Schierenbeck, T., Riemann, D., Berger, M., & Hornyak, M. (2008). Effect of illicit recreational drugs upon sleep: cocaine, ecstasy and marijuana. *Sleep Medicine Reviews, 12*: 381–389.

Schrader, H., Bovim, G., & Sand, T. (1993). The prevalence of delayed and advanced sleep phase syndromes. *Journal of Sleep Research, 2*(1): 51–55.

Schredl, M., Bohusch, C., Kahl, J., Mader, A., & Somesan, A. (2000). The use of dreams in psychotherapy: a survey of psychotherapists in private practice. *Journal of Psychotherapy Practice and Research, 9*: 81–87.

Schretlen, D. J., & Shapiro, A. M. (2003). A quantitative review of the effects of traumatic brain injury on cognitive functioning. *International Review of Psychiatry, 15*: 341–349.

Shapiro, F., Vogelmann-Sine, S., & Sine, L. F. (1994). Eye movement desensitization and reprocessing: treating trauma and substance abuse. *Journal of Psychoactive Drugs, 26*: 379–391.

Sharpless, B.A., & Barber, J.P. (2011). Lifetime prevalence rates of sleep paralysis: a systematic review. *Sleep Medicine Reviews* 15(5): 311–315.

Sivertsen, B., & Nordhus, I. H. (2007). Management of insomnia in older adults. *British Journal of Psychiatry, 190*: 285–286.

Sivertsen, B., Omvik, S., Pallesen, S., Bjorvatn, B., Havik, O. E., Kvale, G., Nielsen, G. H., & Nordhus, I. H. (2006). Cognitive behavioural therapy *vs* zopiclone for treatment of chronic primary insomnia in older adults. *Journal of the American Medical Association* 295: 2851–2858.

Solms, M. (1997). What is consciousness? *Journal of the American Psychoanalytic Association.* 45: 681–778.

Souders, M. C., Mason, T. B. A., Valladares, O., Bucan, M., Levy, S. E., Mandell, D. S., Weaver, T. E., & Pinto-Martin, J. (2009). Sleep behaviors and sleep quality in children with autism spectrum disorders. *Sleep, 32*: 1566–1578.

Spiegelhalder, K., Espie, C. A., Nissen, C., & Riemann, D. (2008). Sleep-related attentional bias in patients with primary insomnia compared with sleep experts and healthy controls. *Journal of Sleep Research, 17*: 191–196.

Spielman, A.J., Saskin, P., & Thorpy, M.J. (1987). Treatment of chronic insomnia by restriction of time in bed. *Sleep, 10*(1): 45–56.

Tang, N. K. (2009). Cognitive-behavioral therapy for sleep abnormalities of chronic pain patients. *Current Rheumatology Reports, 11*: 451–460.

Tang, N. K., & Harvey, A. G. (2004). Correcting distorted perception of sleep in insomnia: a novel behavioural experiment? *Behaviour Research and Therapy, 42*(1): 27–39.

Thommessen, B., Aarsland, D., Braekhuis, A., Oksengaard, A. R., Engedal, K., & Laake, K. (2002). The psychosocial burden on spouses of the elderly with stroke, dementia and Parkinson's Disease. *International Journal of Geriatric Psychiatry, 17*(1): 78–84.

Thünker, J., & Pietrowsky, R. (2012). Effectiveness of a manualized imagery rehearsal therapy for patients suffering from nightmare disorders with and without a comorbidity of depression or PTSD. *Behaviour Research and Therapy, 50*: 558–564.

Tikotzky, L., & Sadeh, A. (2009). Maternal sleep-related cognitions and infant sleep: a longitudinal study from pregnancy through the 1st year. *Child Development, 80*: 860–874.

Tikotzky, L., & Sadeh, A. (2010). The role of cognitive-behavioral therapy in behavioral childhood insomnia. *Sleep Medicine, 11*: 686–691.

Toh, K. L., Jones, C. R., He, Y., Eide, E. J., Hinz, W. A., Virshup, D. M., Ptácek, L. J., & Fu, Y. H. (2001). An hPer2 phosphorylation site mutation in familial advanced sleep phase syndrome. *Science, 291*: 1040–1043.

Tomfohr, L. M., Schweizer, C. A., Dimsdale, J. E., & Loredo, J. S. (2013). Psychometric characteristics of the Pittsburgh Sleep Quality Index in English speaking non-Hispanic whites and English and Spanish speaking Hispanics of Mexican descent. *Journal of Clinical Sleep Medicine, 9*(1): 61–66.

Trauer, J. M., Qian, M. Y., Doyle, J. S., Rajaratnam, S. M., & Cunnington, D. (2015). Cognitive behavioral therapy for chronic insomnia: A systematic review and meta-analysis. *Annals of Internal Medicine, 163*: 191–204.

Valli, K., Revonsuo, A., Palkas, O., Ismail, K., Ali, K. & Punamaki, R. (2005). The threat simulation theory of the evolutionary function of dreaming: Evidence from dreams of traumatized children. *Consciousness and Cognition, 14*(1): 188–218.

Vallières, A., Ceklic, T., Bastien, C. H., & Espie, C. A. (2013). A preliminary evaluation of the physiological mechanisms of action for sleep restriction therapy. *Sleep Disorders*. Published online 20 November 2013. www.hindawi.com/journals/sd/2013/726372/abs/ [last accessed 20 July 2016].

Van de Castle, R. (1994). *Our Dreaming Mind*. Aquarian Press. London.

van Maanen, A., Meijer, A. M., van der Heijden, K. B., & Oort, F. J. (2015). The effects of light therapy on sleep problems: A systematic review and meta-analysis. *Sleep Medicine Reviews, 29*: 52–62.

Van Someren, E. J. W., Kessler, A., Mirmiran, M., & Swaab, D. F. (1997). Indirect bright light improves circadian rest-activity rhythm disturbances in demented patients. *Biological Psychiatry, 41*: 955–963.

van Straten, A., & Cuijpers, P. (2009). Self-help therapy for insomnia: a meta-analysis. *Sleep Medicine Reviews, 13*(1): 61–71.

Vetrugno, R., Lugaresi, E., Ferini-Strambi, L., & Montagna, P. (2008). Catathrenia (nocturnal groaning): what is it? *Sleep, 31*: 308–309.

Vincent, N., & Walsh, K. (2013). Stepped care for insomnia: an evaluation of implementation in routine practice. *Journal of Clinical Sleep Medicine, 9*: 227–234.

Weaver, L. L. (2015). Effectiveness of work, activities of daily living, education, and sleep interventions for people with autism spectrum disorder: A systematic review. *American Journal Occupational Therapy, 69*: 1–11.

Williams-Buckley, A., Rodrigues, A. J., Jennison, K., Buckley, J., Thurm, A., Sato, S., & Swedo, S. (2010). REM sleep percentage in children with autism compared to children with developmental delay and typical development. *Archives of Pediatric and Adolescent Medicine: 164*: 1032–1037.

Wilson, D. L., Barnes, M., Ellett, L., Permezel, M., Jackson, M., & Crowe, S. F. (2011). Decreased sleep efficiency, increased wake after sleep onset and increased cortical arousals in late pregnancy. *Australian and New Zealand Journal of Obstetric Gynaecology, 51*(1): 38–46.

Wirojanan, J., Jacquemont, S., Diaz, R., Bacalman, S., Anders, T. F., Hagerman, R. J., & Goodlin-Jones, B. L. (2009). The efficacy of melatonin for sleep problems in children with autism, fragile X syndrome, or autism and fragile X syndrome. *Journal of Clinical Sleep Medicine, 5*: 145–150.

Wong, M. Y., Ree, M. J., & Lee, C. W. (2015). Enhancing CBT for chronic insomnia: A randomised clinical trial of additive components of mindfulness or cognitive therapy. *Clinical Psychology and Psychotherapy, 26*.

Woodward, W. C. (2011). Cognitive-behavioral therapy for insomnia in patients with cancer. *Clinical Journal of Oncology Nursing, 15*: E42–E52.

World Health Organization. (1992). *The ICD-10 Classification of Mental and Behavioural Disorders: Clinical Descriptions and Diagnostic Guidelines*. Geneva: World Health Organization.

Xu, J., Wang, L. L., Dammer, E. B., Li, C. B., Xu, G., Chen, S. D., & Wang, G. (2015). Melatonin for sleep disorders and cognition in dementia: a meta-analysis of randomized controlled trials. *American Journal of Alzheimers Disease and Other Dementias, 30*: 439–447.

Yalom, I. D. (2002). *The Gift of Therapy: Reflections on Being a Therapist.* London: Pikatus.

Yazaki, M., Shirakawa, S., Okawa, M., & Takahashi, K. (1999). Demography of sleep disturbances associated with circadian rhythm disorders in Japan. *Psychiatry and Clinical Neuroscience, 53*: 267–268.

Ye, Y.-Y., Zhang, Y.-F., Chen, J., Liu, J., Li, X.-J., & Liu, Y.-Z. (2015). Internet-based cognitive behavioral therapy for insomnia (ICBT-i) improves comorbid anxiety and depression—a meta-analysis of randomized controlled trials. *PLoSONE, 10*: e0142258.

Young, T., Rabago, D., Zgierska, A., Austin, D., & Finn, L. (2003). Objective and subjective sleep quality in premenopausal, perimenopausal, and postmenopausal women in the Wisconsin Sleep Cohort Study. *Sleep, 26*: 667–672.

INDEX

191